100 Questions & Answers About Valvular Heart Disease

Ramdas G. Pai, MD
Director of Cardiac Imaging Center
Director Heart Valve Center
Loma Linda University Medical Center
Loma Linda, CA

Padmini Varadarajan, MD
Assistant Professor of Medicine
Loma Linda University Medical Center
Loma Linda, CA

D1089561

JONES AND BARTLETT PUBLISHERS
Sudbury, Massachusetts
BOSTON   TORONTO   LONDON   SINGAPORE

World Headquarters

Jones and Bartlett Publishers
40 Tall Pine Drive
Sudbury, MA 01776
978-443-5000
info@jbpub.com
www.jbpub.com

Jones and Bartlett Publishers
Canada
6339 Ormindale Way
Mississauga, Ontario L5V 1J2
CANADA

Jones and Bartlett Publishers
International
Barb House, Barb Mews
London W6 7PA
United Kingdom

Jones and Bartlett's books and products are available through most bookstores and online book-sellers. To contact Jones and Bartlett Publishers directly, call 800-832-0034, fax 978-443-8000, or visit our website, www.jbpub.com.

Substantial discounts on bulk quantities of Jones and Bartlett's publications are available to corporations, professional associations, and other qualified organizations. For details and specific discount information, contact the special sales department at Jones and Bartlett via the above contact information or send an email to specialsales@jbpub.com.

The authors, editor, and publisher have made every effort to provide accurate information. However, they are not responsible for errors, omissions, or for any outcomes related to the use of the contents of this book and take no responsibility for the use of the products and procedures described. Treatments and side effects described in this book may not be applicable to all people; likewise, some people may require a dose or experience a side effect that is not described herein. Drugs and medical devices are discussed that may have limited availability controlled by the Food and Drug Administration (FDA) for use only in a research study or clinical trial. Research, clinical practice, and government regulations often change the accepted standard in this field. When consideration is being given to use of any drug in the clinical setting, the health care provider or reader is responsible for determining FDA status of the drug, reading the package insert, and reviewing prescribing information for the most up-to-date recommendations on dose, precautions, and contraindications, and determining the appropriate usage for the product. This is especially important in the case of drugs that are new or seldom used.

Cover Credits
Top photo (man): © Galina Barskaya/ShutterStock, Inc.
Bottom photo (woman): © Elena Elisseeva/ShutterStock, Inc.

Production Credits
Executive Publisher: Christopher Davis
Acquisitions Editor: Janice Hackenberg
Editorial Assistant: Jessica Acox
Production Director: Amy Rose
Production Editor: Daniel Stone
Associate Marketing Manger: Llana Goddess

Manufacturing Buyer: Therese Connell
Composition: Northeast Compositors, Inc.
Cover Design: Jonathan Ayotte
Printing and Binding: Malloy, Inc.
Cover Printing: Malloy, Inc.

Library of Congress Cataloging-in-Publication Data
Pai, Ramdas G.
   100 questions & answers about valvular heart disease / Ramdas Pai, Padmini
Varadarajan.
      p. cm.
   Includes bibliographical references and index.
   ISBN-13: 978-0-7637-5387-0
   ISBN-10: 0-7637-5387-4
   1. Heart valves--Diseases--Popular works. 2. Heart
valves--Diseases--Miscellanea. I. Varadarajan, Padmini. II. Title. III.
Title: 100 questions and answers about valvular heart disease. IV. Title:
One hundred questions & answers about valvular heart disease.
   RC685.V2P35 2008
   616.1'25--dc22
                                    2008017269

6048

Printed in the United States of America
12 11 10 09 08   10 9 8 7 6 5 4 3 2 1

We would like to dedicate this book to our patients who taught us, trusted us, and gave us the privilege of taking care of them; to our families who supported us; and to our teachers who mentored us.

Contents

Questions 1–6 cover basic information about the structure and function of the heart and valves, such as:

- Where is the heart located, and what are its components?
- Why are the heart valves important?
- What happens when the valves malfunction?

Questions 7–53 provide information about a variety of sources of valvular heart disease and how to recognize it, including:

- What is valve prolapse?
- What are the mechanisms of degenerative valve disease?
- Which valve or valves are affected by ischemic valve disease?

Questions 54–57 provide information on when and how to intervene, with answers to such questions as:

- What needs to be done if there is a valve problem?
- What are the general guidelines for surgical intervention?
- Who needs endocarditis prophylaxis?

Questions 58–67 explore a number of surgical approaches, valve options, and anticoagulation issues, like:

- What are the types of surgery for valve disorders?
- What are the long-term outcomes with artificial valves?
- What are the complications of warfarin therapy?

Most lay people think of heart disease merely as a problem of cholesterol buildup, plaque formation, and development of heart attack. There is little awareness of disorders associated with malfunction of the four valves in the heart chambers that permit blood movement in a forward direction (from one chamber to the other, e.g. left atrium to left ventricle). Many of these valve disorders are silent until the more advanced stages, when symptoms develop. Although the valve disorders may be diagnosed with help of the stethoscope, a more accurate assessment is provided by cardiac ultrasound (echocardiography). Even as medications may help mitigate some of the symptoms of advanced valve disease, the more definitive treatment consists of surgical repair or replacement of diseased valves.

Drs. Ramdas Pai and Padmini Varadarajan have performed a valuable service in this book, aptly titled *100 Questions & Answers About Valvular Heart Disease*. The information is valuable and timely, since incidence of valvular disease is on the rise with increasing life expectancy. An interested reader will find answers to many of his or her own questions relative to valvular disease, making this book an excellent starting point in collecting information. When surgery is being considered, it is important to gather information about the expertise and track record of the specific surgeon. Not all surgeons and not all hospitals are equal in this regard. All cardiothoracic surgeons claim to be able to repair valves, but in reality only a few are able to do it consistently well. The prospective patient must explore Web sites and ask appropriate questions to get the best opportunity for successful surgery.

I highly recommend this informative book written in a lucid style.

Pravin M. Shah, MD, MACC
Chair, Medical Director
Hoag Heart Valve Center
One Hoag Drive
Newport Beach, CA

Both of us are cardiologists with special interests in taking care of patients with valvular heart disease and in cardiac imaging. We have had the privilege of taking care of patients with simple, as well as complex, valvular problems over the last 15–20 years. Many times the significant valvular problem was part of a complex puzzle of weakening of the heart muscle, coronary artery disease, advanced age, and other disease processes in the body impacting both genesis of symptoms and management decisions. Solving these puzzles has been both challenging and gratifying. We have learned immensely from our patients because of their questions and concerns. Education in which the patient is a partner in the management process is a critical component of management of chronic disease processes. This partnership results in the best success rate. Hence, we came up with the common questions the patients have generally asked us, answers to the concerns they have, and types of information patients with valvular problems should understand to best manage their problems. Our goal is to empower the patients with a thorough knowledge of their problems.

We deeply appreciate the opportunity given to us by Jones and Bartlett to publish this work and make it available to patients and caregivers who can use it as an educational tool. We specifically want to thank Ms. Janice Hackenberg and Mr. Chris Davis for their interest in our work, as well as for their support.

The book is divided into multiple sections addressing basics, general aspects of the disease processes, surgical treatments, and specific valvular problems, with illustrative images. The answer to Question 100 lists where to find additional information. The glossary of terms should be helpful while navigating the book. The index can direct the readers to specific questions they may have in mind. However, a complete reading of the book would be helpful for patients as it would give a good overview of the valvular problems and their management.

We greatly appreciate the opportunity to be of assistance to our patients and also their caregivers.

Ramdas G. Pai, MD, FACC, FRCP (Edin)
Padmini Varadarajan, MD, FACC

PART ONE

The Basics

What are heart valves, and what do they do?

Where is the heart located, and what
are its components?

How does the blood flow through the heart?

More ...

STRUCTURE AND FUNCTION OF THE HEART

1. What are heart valves, and what do they do?

Valves are flaplike structures that allow blood to flow in only one direction. There are four heart valves. These are mitral, aortic, tricuspid, and **pulmonary valves**. The moving structures of the valves are called leaflets. The **mitral valve** has two leaflets and the other three valves have three leaflets each. There is also a rudimentary valve, the **eustachian valve**, between the **inferior vena cava** and the right **atrium**, which has no functional significance.

It is important that the valves allow blood flow only in the forward direction, e.g. from left atrium to left ventricle, without any impediment, and that there is no significant backflow. Impediment to flow due to narrowing is called stenosis, and backflow is called regurgitation. Both can be detrimental to **cardiac** function.

2. Where is the heart located, and what are its components?

The heart is located behind the left side of the chest and is the size of a fist. It has four chambers and four valves and is connected to two great arteries (the **aorta** and the **pulmonary artery**), two **vena cavae** (superior and inferior), and four **pulmonary veins** (two from the

---

Valve

A structure made of two or three leaflets designed to allow blood to flow in one direction only. There are four valves inside the heart—mitral, aortic, tricuspid, and pulmonary.

Pulmonary valve

The trileaflet valve between the right ventricle and the pulmonary artery.

Mitral valve

A bileaflet valve separating the left atrium and left ventricle.

Eustachian valve

A vestigial valve between the inferior vena cava and the right atrium with no known functions in adult life. In the intrauterine life, this directs umbilical vein flow into the left atrium through the patent foramen ovale.

Inferior vena cava

A large vein that drains impure blood from the lower part of the body into the right atrium.

Atrium

One of two upper chambers that receives blood; the right atrium receives blood from the body and the left atrium receives it from the lungs.

right lung and two from the left lung). The pumping chambers are called **ventricles**, and the receiving chambers are called atria (Figure 1). The right side of the heart receives blood from the body and delivers blood to the lung for oxygenation. The left side receives **oxygenated** blood from the lungs and pumps to the entire body.

3. How does the blood flow through the heart?

As shown in Figure 2, the oxygen-depleted blood comes to the right atrium through inferior and **superior vena cavae**, which are large veins collecting impure or **deoxygenated** blood from the lower and upper parts of the body, respectively. From the right atrium, the blood flows into the right ventricle through the **tricuspid valve**, which allows blood to flow in this direction only. The right ventricle pumps blood into the lungs through the pulmonary valve and artery during **systole** to be oxygenated. From the lungs, the oxygenated blood flows through the four pulmonary veins into the left atrium. From there, it flows into the left ventricle through the mitral valve. The left ventricle pumps blood to the entire body during systole through the **aortic valve**.

4. Why are the heart valves important?

The heart valves allow blood to flow in one direction only, or are unidirectional valves. For example, the tri-

The Basics

Cardiac
Related to the heart.

Aorta
The artery transporting blood from the left ventricle to the rest of the body through its various branches.

Pulmonary artery
The artery that transports blood from the right ventricle to the lungs.

Vena cava
One of the two large veins that drain impure blood from the body into the right atrium.

Pulmonary vein
A thin walled blood vessel that brings oxygenated blood from the lungs into the left atrium. There are four pulmonary veins, two from each lung.

Ventricle
Lower chamber of the heart that pumps blood into an artery. The left ventricle pumps into the aorta. The right ventricle pumps into the pulmonary artery, which takes blood into the lungs to be oxygenated.

Oxygenated
Replenished with oxygen, e.g., blood that is replenished with oxygen by the lungs.

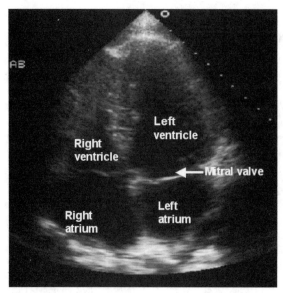

(a)

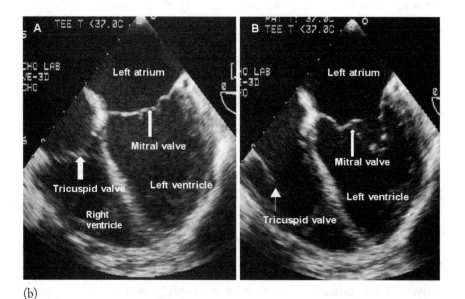

(b)

Figure 1 Ultrasound or echocardiographic examination of the heart showing the 4 cardiac chambers. Figure 1A is a transthoracic image where images are obtained from the surface of the chest. Figure 1B is a transesophageal image where a small tube is introduced into the food pipe to obtain the images. Transesophageal echocardiography gives higher resolution images and better visualization of the valves, left atrium and the aorta.

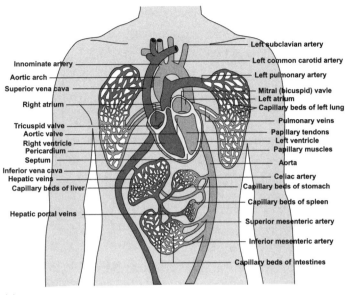

(a)

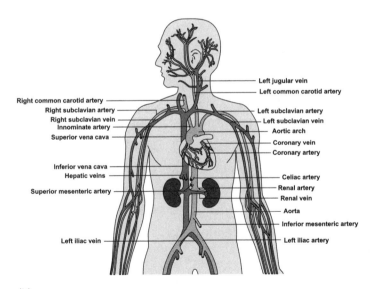

(b)

Figure 2   Schematic of circulation: Illustrations showing blood circulation, and how the various parts of the circulation are related to each other.
Redrawn courtesy of Dr. Kimball from Kimball's Biology Pages, http://biology-pages.info/.

cuspid valve allows blood to flow from the right atrium to the right ventricle with no impediment and prevents blood from leaking back into the right atrium when the right ventricle contracts in order to eject blood into the pulmonary artery. Similarly, the pulmonary valve prevents blood from leaking back into the right ventricle when the right ventricle relaxes in order to receive blood from the right atrium. The mitral valve is a unidirectional valve between the left atrium and the left ventricle, preventing blood from leaking back into the left atrium and hence back into the lungs when the left ventricle contracts or squeezes blood into the aorta. The aortic valve prevents blood from leaking back from aorta into the left ventricle. In general, the main function of the valves is to ascertain that blood flows in a forward direction only.

5. What can go wrong with the valves?

A variety of things can happen to the valves. Because of **inflammation** or calcium deposits, they can get narrower or blocked; this is called **stenosis** (Figure 3). They can also get leaky; this is called **regurgitation** (Figure 4). Infection of the heart valve is called **endocarditis,** which can cause fever, severe illness, and destruction of the valve (Figure 5). The heart valves can be congenitally malformed as well.

6. What happens when the valves malfunction?

When the valves malfunction, what happens depends upon the type of malfunction and location of the valve. For example, if the mitral valve narrows or blocks

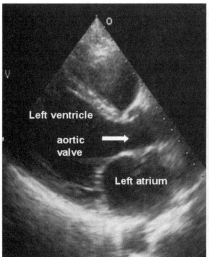

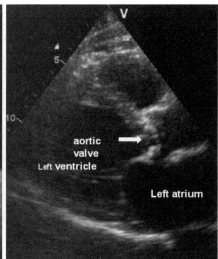

(a)

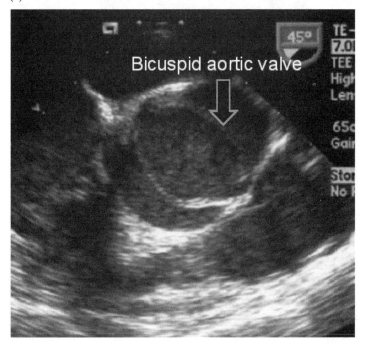

(b)

Figure 3   Aortic valve as seen by echocardiography cutting through the valve during systole when the valve is in open position. (a) Normal trileaflet valve with normal opening during systole and narrowed or stenosed valve due to calcification. (b) A bicuspid valve with 2 leaflets which occurs in 2% of the population.

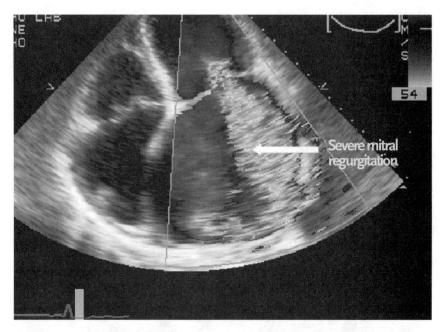

Figure 4   Leaky or regurgitatnt mitral valve: the large blue jet is the regurgitant jet seen in the left atrium or the receiving upper chamber.

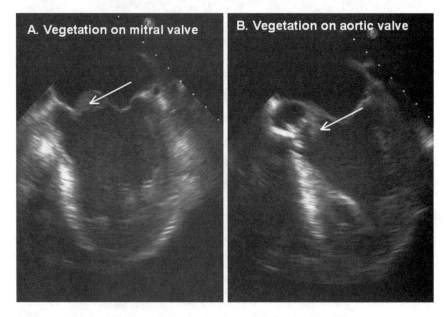

Figure 5   Endocarditis, which refers to infection of the heart valves. In this image, infected masses called vegetations are seen on the mitral and aortic valves.

(**mitral stenosis**), the pressure builds upstream in the left atrium and the lungs; this causes shortness of breath, enlargement of the left atrium, and increase in the pressure inside the lung arteries. A leaky mitral valve (**mitral regurgitation**) not only increases the size and pressure in the left atrium, but increases the amount of work the left ventricle has to perform; hence, the left ventricle enlarges and ultimately weakens. Aortic valve stenosis makes it difficult for the left ventricle to squeeze blood through the narrowed aortic valve. In an effort to do this, the left ventricle has to generate a higher pressure and develops thicker walls (**hypertrophy**). This may ultimately lead to damage to the heart muscle, and its weakening leads to **heart failure**.

Stenosis
Narrowing of a valve or a blood vessel.

Regurgitation
Leaky valve.

Endocarditis
Inflammation of the valve or inner lining of the heart generally due to infection such as streptococcus or staphylococcus.

Mitral stenosis
Narrowed mitral valve such that the left atrial pressure rises in order to push blood forward, from the left atrium to the left ventricle.

Mitral regurgitation
Leaky mitral valve such that blood leaks back from the left ventricle into the left atrium.

Hypertrophy
Thickening of the wall of the heart due to more muscle mass.

Heart failure
A situation where demand on the heart exceeds its capacity. It generally occurs due to weakening of the heart muscle or a severe valve problem. Manifestations include shortness of breath, swelling in the legs, fatigue, and swollen neck veins.

The Basics

PART TWO

Causes, Symptoms, and Diagnosis

What are some of the causes of valvular heart disease?

What causes rheumatic fever?

What age groups are affected by rheumatic fever?

More . . .

7. What are some of the causes of valvular heart disease?

The valve can be damaged because of rheumatic fever, infections (endocarditis), wear and tear changes (**degenerative** changes), or rarely because of drugs (e.g., **Fen-phen** intake for obesity). The mitral valve can also leak because of mitral valve prolapse or ischemic heart disease. The aortic valve can also narrow or leak because of **congenital** abnormalities (e.g., **bicuspid** aortic valve). The aortic valve can leak because of enlargement of the aorta (**aneurysm**) as well. Heart attack or coronary artery disease can deform the mitral valve and can cause it to leak. A dilated heart can do the same thing as well. An aortic aneurysm can cause **aortic regurgitation**. Sometimes blunt trauma to the chest can result in rupture of the valves, causing a leak. The most commonly involved valve in blunt trauma is the tricuspid valve.

RHEUMATIC HEART DISEASE
8. What causes rheumatic fever?

Rheumatic fever is a condition causing inflammation of the body's connective tissues, especially those of the heart, joints, brain, or skin. Rheumatic heart disease occurs after an attack of rheumatic fever, caused by streptococcal throat infection. This condition is not common to the industrialized nations, but it is a problem in developing countries. Generally, the rheumatic fever occurs 2–3 weeks after a streptococcal throat

Degenerative

Change produced by wear and tear.

Fen-Phen

A combination of weight-loss drugs used in the 1990s that caused valvular problems. This drug was taken off the market with a large class-action lawsuit.

Congenital

Something one is born with.

Bicuspid

A valve made of two valve leaflets.

Aneurysm

Abnormal dilatation of an artery or a cardiac chamber. A dilated blood vessel increases the risk of rupture.

Aortic regurgitation

A leaky aortic valve such that blood leaks back from the aorta to the left ventricle.

infection, causing joint pain or swelling and rarely skin lesions. It also causes inflammation in the heart and abnormal involuntary movements called chorea. Joint problems are temporary, but heart problems could be permanent, hence the saying, "rheumatic fever licks the joints, but bites the heart."

9. What age groups are affected by rheumatic fever?

Acute rheumatic fever can affect any age group, but it usually occurs in children between the ages of 5 and 15 years. Once rheumatic heart disease has affected the heart valves, it lasts a lifetime.

10. Which valves are commonly affected by rheumatic fever?

Valves most commonly affected by rheumatic fever are the mitral and aortic valves, in that order. Rarely, tricuspid and pulmonic valves can be affected as well. The inflammation causes the valve leaflets to thicken and stick to each other. The leaflets can get deformed and calcify. This can cause valve stenosis, regurgitation, or both.

11. What are the symptoms of rheumatic fever?

During an acute attack of rheumatic fever, symptoms vary greatly. Symptoms of rheumatic fever appear about 2 weeks after the onset of an untreated strep

Rheumatic fever

Fever that may occur after streptococcal infections, resulting in joint pains, skin lesions, and inflammation of the heart. Inflammation of the heart results in valvular problems.

Joint problems are temporary, but heart problems could be permanent, hence the saying, "rheumatic fever licks the joints, but bites the heart."

throat. Apart from sore throat, and fever, the child will have a painful, swollen red joint (the fever affects one joint at a time, causing no permanent damage, and it migrates to another joint). Short-lived skin rashes may occur.

12. What are the symptoms of rheumatic heart disease?

Damage to the heart valves is not immediately noticeable. A damaged heart valve either does not open fully (referred to as valve stenosis) or close (valve regurgitation). Initially, the patient might not experience any symptoms. As the valve damage becomes more severe, symptoms of shortness of breath, decreased exercise tolerance, **palpitations**, swelling of the feet, and finally **congestive heart failure** occur. This is a condition where the heart enlarges and is not able to pump blood.

Palpitations

Feeling one's own heartbeat. This could be either benign or abnormal.

Congestive heart failure

See heart failure.

13. How does one diagnose rheumatic fever and rheumatic heart disease clinically?

During an acute rheumatic fever, a patient has swollen painful joints, and a skin rash can be seen. Examination of the heart with the stethoscope may not reveal anything abnormal. When rheumatic heart disease occurs, the physician can hear abnormal heart sounds and **murmurs**.

Murmur

A noise produced by flowing blood that can be heard with a stethoscope. Some noises could be normal, but louder ones and diastolic ones are generally abnormal.

14. What diagnostic tests are helpful in the diagnosis of rheumatic heart disease?

The most helpful test is a **transthoracic echocardiogram**. **Cardiac catheterization** may be helpful to evaluate valves and measure pressures. Rarely, a **Holter monitor** may be helpful to evaluate for abnormal rhythms.

Echocardiogram: This test utilizes sound waves for examination of the heart valves. With rheumatic heart disease of the mitral valve, calcification of the various parts of the mitral valve can be seen, causing either a restricted opening or an abnormal closure (Figure 6). Pressures across the valve can also be calculated using **Doppler** technology to quantify the severity of the valve stenosis. Valvular regurgitation can be assessed using color flow imaging. Similarly, rheumatic heart disease of the aortic valve causes abnormal calcification of the valve, causing stenosis or regurgitation.

Cardiac catheterization: This is carried out through the femoral (groin) artery and vein, wherein catheters are floated up to the heart and pressures are recorded in the left ventricle (left bottom chamber). It is also carried out through a vein in the groin wherein pressures are recorded in the right atrium (top right chamber), right ventricle (bottom right chamber) and pulmonary artery and pulmonary wedge pressure which is a surrogate of pressures in the left atrium (top left chamber). The severity of valve leakage can be ascertained by abnormal pressure waves in the top left chamber (left atrium).

Transthoracic echocardiogram

A standard, non-invasive echocardiogram where a transducer records the sound wave echoes of the heart as they reflect off internal structures.

Cardiac catheterization

Inserting a catheter into the heart through a peripheral artery or a vein to record the pressures or obtain an angiogram or intervene to fix a lesion.

Holter monitor

A device for continuous monitoring of the heartbeat to detect arrhythmia. Generally, this is worn for 24-48 hrs and when symptoms occur, the patient can store the recording by pressing a button.

Doppler

An ultrasound examination of the heart based on Doppler principle. This allows visualization of flow and measurement of blood flow velocities.

Causes, Symptoms, and Diagnosis

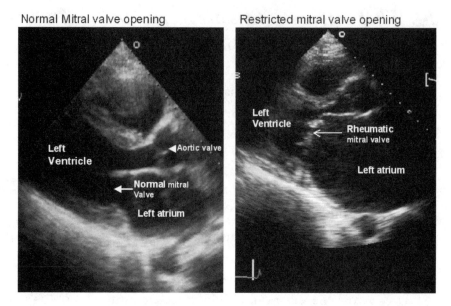

Figure 6 Echocardiogram showing normal opening of the mitral valve and mitral stenosis which is narrowing of the valve. Mitral valve opens in diastole.

Holter: A 24-hour Holter monitor can evaluate palpitations or abnormally rapid heartbeat. This is a continuous recording of the patient's heart rhythm as he or she carries out his or her daily activities. Abnormal rhythms are recorded on the tape and analyzed at a later date. The Holter may fail to capture an abnormal rhythm if it does not occur daily. In that case, an event monitor is used to detect abnormal rhythms. The patient can be fitted with an event recorder to be worn for several weeks. When the patient experiences a palpitation, an event button can be pressed to record the heart rhythm during that episode.

15. Can rheumatic heart disease be prevented?

The best method of preventing rheumatic heart disease is to prevent rheumatic fever from occurring. Treating strep throat with penicillin or other antibiotics can prevent acute rheumatic fever. People who have already developed rheumatic fever are susceptible to heart damage. That is why they are given monthly or daily antibiotic treatment until a certain age or maybe for life. Patients with rheumatic heart disease are at increased risk of developing infection of the heart's lining or valves.

PROLAPSE
16. What is valve prolapse?

Prolapse of the valve means to flop backwards, causing the valve not to close fully. A normal mitral valve consists of two thin leaflets, located between the left atrium (top left chamber) and the left ventricle (main pumping chamber) of the heart. Mitral valve leaflets, shaped like parachutes, are attached to the inner wall of the left ventricle by a series of strings called chordae. When the ventricles contract, the mitral valve leaflets close snugly and prevent the backflow of blood from the left ventricle into the left atrium. When the ventricles relax, the valves open to allow oxygenated blood from the lungs to fill the left ventricle.

In patients with mitral valve prolapse, the mitral apparatus (valve leaflets and chordae) becomes affected by a

Prolapse
Excessive systolic motion of a cardiac valve due to loss of support.

17

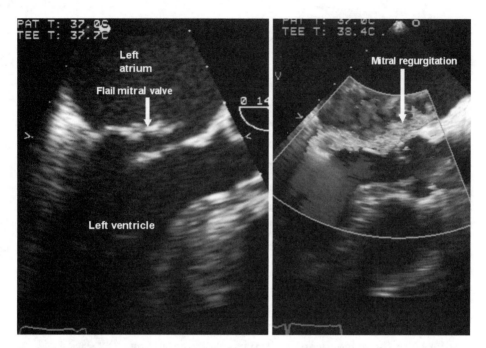

Figure 7 Echocardiogram of a flail mitral valve which refers to torn chordae tendinae such that the valve flops back into the left atrium causing severe mitral regurgitation.

Myxomatous

Thickened, fluffy, weaker tissue as may occur in mitral valve prolapse.

process called **myxomatous** degeneration. In myxomatous degeneration, the structural protein collagen forms abnormally and causes thickening, enlargement, and elongation of the leaflets and chordae. When the ventricles contract, the elongated leaflets prolapse (flop backwards) into the left atrium, sometimes allowing leakage of blood through the valve opening (mitral regurgitation) (Figure 7).

17. What are the risk factors for mitral valve prolapse?

The mitral valve prolapse (MVP) syndrome has a strong hereditary tendency, although the exact cause is unknown. Affected family members are often tall and thin, with long arms and fingers and straight backs. It is seen most commonly in women from 20 to 40 years old, but it also occurs in men.

18. Which valves are most commonly affected?

The most common valve to prolapse is mitral, rarely the tricuspid valve. The aortic valve can prolapse as well.

19. What are the symptoms of a prolapsed valve?

Initially, when the prolapse is mild, there might not be any symptoms. Fatigue is the most common complaint, although the reason for fatigue is not understood. Patients with mitral valve prolapse may have imbalances in their autonomic nervous system, which regulates heart rate and breathing. Such imbalances may cause inadequate blood oxygen delivery to the working muscles during exercise, thereby causing fatigue. Palpitations are sensations of fast or irregular heartbeats. In most patients with mitral valve prolapse, palpitations are harmless. In very rare cases, potentially serious heart rhythm abnormalities may underlie palpitations, which require further evaluation and treatment. Patients often report sharp chest pains, which is rarely due to **angina** (chest pain due to decreased oxygen supply to the heart muscle). **Migraine** headaches are often linked with mitral valve prolapse. **Strokes** can occasionally occur in patients with mitral valve prolapse, probably due to platelets aggregating on the thickened leaflets. When the prolapse becomes severe,

Angina

Chest pain due to lack of blood supply to the heart muscle. This generally occurs due to a blockage in the coronary artery. Generally the chest pain is exertional.

Migraine

A throbbing headache thought to be related to excessive dilation of the blood vessels in the brain due to some circulating substance. There is an association with patent foramen ovale and mitral valve prolapse.

Stroke

Damage to part of the brain due a blockage in the artery or bleeding.

patients might experience shortness of breath, decreased exercise capacity, and finally, congestive heart failure.

20. How can prolapse be diagnosed clinically?

With a stethoscope, physicians can often hear a clicking sound soon after the main pumping chamber (left ventricle) begins to contract (during systole). This clicking sound reflects the tightening of the abnormal valve leaflets against the pressure load of the left ventricle. If there is associated leakage of blood due to the incomplete closure of the valve, a whooshing sound (murmur) can be heard after the clicking sound.

21. What diagnostic tests are useful in the diagnosis of valve prolapse?

Echocardiography

Examination of the heart using ultrasound. One can obtain images of the heart and examine blood flows.

Ultrasound

Sound wave above the hearing range (> 20,000 Hz) used to perform echocardiography.

Echocardiography, catheterization, and a Holter test are used to diagnose valve prolapse.

*Echocardiography (**ultrasound** of the heart):* This is the most useful test for detecting mitral valve prolapse. It can measure the degree of prolapse, and the severity of valve leakage. It can also help in determining the effect of valve leakage on the function of the ventricle. Valve infection (endocarditis) is a rare but serious complication of mitral valve prolapse, which can be detected by ultrasound examination of the heart.

Cardiac catheterization: This is carried out through the femoral (groin) artery and vein, wherein catheters are floated up to the heart and pressures are recorded in the left ventricle (left bottom chamber). It is also carried out through a vein in the groin, wherein pressures are recorded in the right atrium (top right chamber), right ventricle (bottom right chamber), and pulmonary artery and pulmonary capillary wedge pressure which is a surrogate of pressures in the left atrium (top left chamber). The severity of valve leakage can be ascertained by abnormal pressure waves in the top left chamber (left atrium).

Holter: A 24-hour Holter monitor can evaluate palpitations or abnormally rapid heartbeat. This is a continuous recording of the patient's heart rhythm as he carries out his or her daily activities. Abnormal rhythms are recorded on the tape and analyzed at a later date. The Holter may fail to capture an abnormal rhythm if it does not occur daily. In that case, an event monitor is used to detect abnormal rhythms. The patient can be fitted with an event recorder to be worn for several weeks. When the patient experiences a palpitation, an event button can be pressed to record the heart rhythm during that episode.

DEGENERATIVE VALVE DISEASE
22. What is degenerative valve disease?

Degenerative valve disease commonly affects the aortic and the mitral valves. Degeneration of the aortic valve commonly involves calcium buildup in the valve, leading to incomplete opening of the valve. Degenerative disease of the mitral valve involves myxomatous changes of the mitral valve leaflets and their supporting structures, the **chordae tendinae**. This condition

Chordae tendinae
Stringlike structures that support mitral and tricuspid valves.

usually leads to incomplete valve closure. Mitral valve prolapse is a type of myxomatous valve disease. The tissue of the mitral valve leaflets and chordae are abnormally stretchy, so that as the heart beats, the mitral valve bows or flops back into the left atrium. Degenerative mitral valve disease can also occur due to calcium buildup in the mitral valve attachment (**annulus**).

Annulus

A fibrous structure to which the valve leaflets are attached; it serves as a hinge.

23. What age groups are affected by degenerative valve disease?

The age groups affected depend on whether the disease is aortic or mitral.

Calcium buildup that occurs in a trileaflet aortic valve (a normal aortic valve has three leaflets), leads to incomplete opening of the valve. The effects are usually seen in people aged 70 years and older. Calcification of a bicuspid aortic valve (two of the three cusps are fused) usually occurs in younger patients.

Myxomatous degeneration of the mitral valve can affect any age group. It is more common in women. Degenerative mitral valve disease due to calcification usually occurs in older people and in those with kidney failure.

24. What are the mechanisms of degenerative valve disease?

For degenerative aortic valve disease, the process involved in calcification is thought to be similar to atherosclerosis (hardening of the blood vessels due to cholesterol deposition), lipid deposition, activation of scavenger cells, and bone-forming cells.

Microscopic examinations of myxomatous tissues have shown that the mitral leaflets and chordae have disorganized, fragmented collagen and elastic fibers, as well as an abnormal accumulation of glycosaminoglycans (GAGs). GAGs are particular types of carbohydrates that have diverse structural and regulatory roles in connective tissues. In heart valves, for example, it is thought that certain GAGs provide lubrication between the valve layers and allow for recovery from compressive stresses, among other functions.

25. What are the symptoms of degenerative valve disease?

The symptoms of degenerative aortic valve disease are due to an incomplete opening of the aortic valve. Initially, there may be no symptoms. As the valve gets narrower, patients can experience shortness of breath (**dyspnea**) initially with activity and then may progress to symptoms at rest. Patients also can experience chest pain or angina with exertion due to inadequate blood supply to the thickened heart muscle. Finally, this may lead to heart failure.

Dyspnea
Shortness of breath. *See* paroxysmal nocturnal dyspnea.

Degenerative mitral valve disease symptoms are the same as those for mitral valve prolapse (see question 19).

26. How is degenerative valve disease diagnosed clinically?

A physician listening with a stethoscope can hear abnormal heart sounds or murmurs of the aortic or mitral valve. When heart failure sets in, physicians can determine if the pressure is high inside the heart by listening to the lungs and looking at neck veins.

27. What tests are useful in the diagnosis?

Echocardiography (ultrasound of the heart) is the most useful test in detecting aortic valve disease. Using echocardiography, the physician can assess the degree of calcification of the aortic valve, the severity of valve disease (incomplete closure or opening), and the pressures across the valves and in the heart.

Echocardiography, cardiac catheterization, and a Holter monitor are useful for diagnosing mitral valve disease.

Echocardiography (ultrasound of the heart): This is the most useful test for detecting mitral valve prolapse. It can measure the degree of prolapse and the severity of valve leakage. It can also help in determining the effect of valve leakage on the function of the ventricle. Valve infection (endocarditis) is a rare but serious complication of mitral valve prolapse, which can be detected by ultrasound examination of the heart.

Cardiac catheterization: This is carried out through the femoral (groin) artery and vein, wherein catheters are floated up to the heart and pressures are recorded in the left ventricle (left bottom chamber). It is also carried out through a vein in the groin wherein pressures are recorded in the right atrium (top right chamber), right ventricle (bottom right chamber), and pulmonary artery and pulmonary capillary wedge pressure which is a surrogate of pressures in the left atrium (top left chamber). The severity of valve leakage can be ascertained by abnormal pressure waves in the top left chamber (left atrium).

Holter monitor: A 24-hour Holter monitor can evaluate palpitations or abnormally rapid heartbeat. This is a continuous recording of the patient's heart rhythm as he or she carries out their daily activities. Abnormal rhythms are recorded on a tape and analyzed at a later date. A Holter monitor may fail to capture an abnormal rhythm if it does not occur daily. In that case, an event monitor is used to detect abnormal rhythms. The patient can be fitted with an event recorder to be worn for several weeks. When the patient experiences a palpitation, an event button can be pressed to record the heart rhythm during that episode.

ISCHEMIC CAUSES OF VALVULAR HEART DISEASE

28. What is ischemic valve disease?

Valvular problems caused by ischemic heart disease, i.e., problems from blockages in the coronary artery, are called ischemic valve disease. Ischemic valve disease occurs in the setting of a heart attack which causes weakening of the heart muscle, thereby causing it to dilate.

29. Which valve or valves are affected by ischemic valve disease?

Usually the mitral valve is affected in the setting of **ischemia**. Aortic and pulmonary valves are not affected. The tricuspid valve can be affected because of

Ischemia
Reduced blood supply causing lack of oxygen to the tissues.

a right ventricular **infarction**, a heart attack, or high pressures in the pulmonary arteries causing a stress on the tricuspid valve.

30. What is the mechanism of ischemic mitral valve disease?

Ischemic mitral regurgitation (IMR) is a common complication of coronary artery disease caused by partial or complete obstruction of one or more coronary arteries. By definition, patients with IMR have structurally normal valve leaflets and chordae but valvular incompetence usually occurs as a complication of regional or global left ventricular dysfunction. Due to loss of contractility in the left ventricular walls, there is outward displacement of the **papillary muscle**, which leads to inadequate closure of the mitral valve leaflets (Figure 8). This leads to incomplete closure and mitral regurgitation (backward flow of blood into the left

Ischemic mitral regurgitation

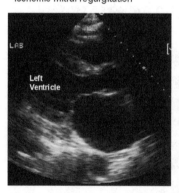 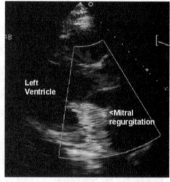

Figure 8 **An echocardiogram of a patient with ischemic mitral regurgitation. Note that the mitral valve is prevented from closing because of pull on it towards the left ventricle.**

atrium when the left ventricle contracts). Ischemic mitral regurgitation is a form of functional mitral regurgitation.

In the acute setting, ischemic mitral valve disease can occur as a mechanical complication in the setting of a heart attack. This is usually seen between 2 and 5 days after a heart attack. The posterior papillary muscle, which has only one arterial blood supply, can get necrosed or damaged. This leads to inadequate support for the mitral valve, causing the valve to prolapse into the left atrium. Often the ruptured papillary muscle can be seen coiling in the left atrium. This occurs commonly when the right coronary artery is blocked.

Often the rup-tured papil-lary muscle can be seen coiling in the left atrium.

31. What are the age groups affected?

Usually people who are at risk for heart disease are affected. Generally these patients are older and may have risk factors for coronary artery disease such as a family history of ischemic mitral valve disease, smoking, diabetes, hypertension, or hypercholesterolemia.

32. What is the presentation of ischemic mitral regurgitation?

When ischemic mitral regurgitation occurs in the setting of a heart attack, chest pain and shortness of breath are the most common symptoms. Patients may also experience **arrhythmia**, such as racing of the heart or slow heart rate. In the setting of acute mitral regurgitation with a ruptured papillary muscle, shortness of breath or dyspnea can be the most common initial

Arrhythmia
Abnormal rhythm that may be too slow or too fast. Examples include heart block and atrial fibrillation.

27

symptom. As the left atrium (top left chamber) cannot accommodate all the regurgitant (or backflow) blood, the pressure in that chamber rises very rapidly. This causes the pressure in the lungs to rise and eventually the lungs get flooded with fluid. Such patients may need to be on a respirator to help them breathe.

33. How is ischemic mitral regurgitation diagnosed?

Ischemic mitral regurgitation is suspected when patients have a heart attack. A murmur can be detected by listening with a stethoscope. In the acute stage, when it occurs in conjunction with an acute heart attack, no murmur can be detected.

34. What tests are useful for the diagnosis?

Ischemic mitral regurgitation is diagnosed by using echocardiography or cardiac catheterization.

Echocardiography (ultrasound of the heart): This is the most useful test that helps in the diagnosis of ischemic mitral regurgitation. It can measure the amount of mitral regurgitation or backflow of blood. It can also help in assessing the pressures in the heart. It can help in the assessment of surgical treatment planning.

Cardiac catheterization: This is carried out through the femoral (groin) artery and vein, wherein catheters are floated up to the heart and pressures are recorded in the left ventricle (left bottom chamber). It is also carried out through a vein in the groin wherein pressures are recorded in the right atrium (top right chamber), right ventricle (bottom right chamber), and pulmonary

Causes, Symptoms, and Diagnosis

artery and pulmonary capillary wedge pressure which is a surrogate of pressures in the left atrium (top left chamber). The severity of valve leakage can be ascertained by abnormal pressure waves in the top left chamber (left atrium). At the same time, dye is injected into the right and left coronary artery systems, by which the degree and number of blockages can be diagnosed.

FUNCTIONAL VALVE DISEASE

35. What is functional mitral valve disease and what valves are affectd?

Functional valve disease occurs in the setting of normal leaflets but with some pathology distorting or dilating the left ventricle. This change in ventricular size and shape is called remodeling. Reversing the changes in the ventricle (called **reverse remodeling**) would eliminate the regurgitation. The mitral and tricuspid valves are the most common valves to be affected.

36. What is the pathogenesis of functional valve disease?

Functional mitral valve disease most commonly occurs when the left ventricle enlarges (**dilated cardiomyopathy**). The normal left ventricle shape is elliptical. When it starts to enlarge, it assumes a more spherical shape. When this occurs, it tends to pull the mitral valve apart (called **tethering**) and does not allow it to close completely. This leads to backflow of blood into the top upper chamber (left atrium).

Reverse remodeling

A favorable change in which the heart size gets smaller.

Dilated cardiomyopathy

Heart muscle disease that causes dilation and weakening of the heart muscle leading to heart failure. Outcome is improved by beta-blockers and angiotensin converting enzyme inhibitors.

Tethering

Restricted systolic mobility of valve leaflets because of being pulled down by chordae tendinae.

Functional tricuspid valve disease occurs when the leaflets are normal, but the annulus (the attachment) enlarges. This leads to inadequate leaflet closure causing backflow of blood into the top right chamber. This occurs secondary to right ventricular enlargement and high pulmonary artery pressures.

37. Who is affected by functional mitral valve disease?

Dilated cardiomyopathy can affect any age group. Some forms are familial. Ischemic mitral regurgitation is also a form of functional mitral regurgitation. Ischemic heart disease affects older individuals.

38. What are the symptoms of functional valve disease?

Shortness of breath is the common initial symptom. In severe cases, patients may find it difficult to lie flat in bed at night and may require many pillows to prop up (termed **orthopnea**), may suddenly wake up from bed in the middle of night gasping for air (termed **paroxysmal nocturnal dyspnea**), may experience swelling of their feet, and have racing of the heart.

Orthopnea

Shortness of breath relieved by sitting up; this is a feature of heart failure.

Paroxysmal nocturnal dyspnea

Intermittent shortness of breath that typically wakes the patient up from sleep at night. Is a sign of left-side heart failure.

39. How is it diagnosed?

A cardiologist can hear a murmur by listening with a stethoscope. It is also suspected when patients complain of the aforementioned symptoms. The diagnosis is confirmed by echocardiography. In patients with severe heart failure, severe functional mitral regurgitation can occur without an audible murmur.

40. What tests help in the diagnosis of functional valve disease?

Echocardiography and cardiac catheterization are useful in the diagnosis of functional valve disease.

Echocardiography (ultrasound of the heart): This is the most useful test that helps in the diagnosis of functional mitral and **tricuspid regurgitation**. It can measure the amount of regurgitation or backflow of blood. It can also help in assessing the pressures in the heart. It can help in the assessment of surgical treatment planning.

Cardiac catheterization: This is carried out through the groin, wherein catheters are floated up to the heart through the groin artery or vein. When carried out through an artery, pressures are recorded in the left atrium (top left chamber) and left ventricle (left bottom chamber). When carried out through a vein in the groin, pressures are recorded in the right atrium (top right chamber), right ventricle (bottom right chamber), and pulmonary artery. The severity of valve leakage can be ascertained by abnormal pressure waves in the top left chamber (left atrium) or the right atrium (top right chamber). At the same time, dye is injected into the right and left coronary artery systems, by which the degree and number of blockages can be diagnosed.

INFECTIVE VALVE DISEASE
41. What is an infection of the valve?

Infective endocarditis refers specifically to infection of the inner lining of the heart (**endocardium**), but the

Tricuspid regurgitation

Leaky tricuspid valve such that blood leaks back from the right ventricle into the right atrium.

Endocardium

Inner lining of the heart.

most common location is the heart valve. The infection may also affect the surrounding structures, heart muscle, and any birth defects that involve abnormal connections between the chambers of the heart or its blood vessels. This is a very serious problem, and anybody with a heart valve problem that develops a fever should see his or her physician immediately.

42. What are the forms of infective endocarditis?

There are two forms of infective endocarditis. Acute infective endocarditis develops suddenly and may become life threatening within days. Sub acute infective endocarditis or sub acute bacterial endocarditis, develops gradually and subtly over a period of weeks to several months. This distinction is somewhat artificial as the presentation depends upon the valve involved, type of organism and changes produced in the valves.

43. What are the causes of infective endocarditis?

The agents that cause infective endocarditis are mostly **bacteria**, but **fungi** can be responsible as well. These get introduced into the bloodstream and then lodge on the heart valves, causing an infection. Abnormal valves, congenitally deformed valves, and artificial valves are more prone to be infected. However, some aggressive bacteria can infect normal valves as well. The bacterial or fungal growth on the valve causes an infected mass called **vegetation**. These masses can get

Bacteria

Microorganisms with a cell wall. The body has many bacteria on the skin, oral cavity, and intestines that do not cause any harm. Sometimes they cause harm, such as infection on the heart valves. Examples include streptococci and staphylococci.

Fungus (plural: fungi)

A microorganism that can cause endocarditis.

Vegetation

An inflammatory mass attached to a valve, endocardium, or endothelium. This is most commonly due to an infection and most commonly occurrs on a heart valve.

dislodged and can potentially cause stroke. The infection can destroy the valve, causing severe regurgitation. It can also cause **abscess** and abnormal communications between various parts of the heart.

Abscess
Collection of pus due to bacterial infection.

44. What are the risk factors for infection of the valve?

Risk factors for the infection include congenitally abnormal or deformed valves. The source of infection in most affected individuals is infected gums; hence oral hygiene is very important. Another risk factor in older people is degeneration of the valves, i.e., calcium deposition in the aortic and mitral valves. People who use illicit drugs are at very high risk as they are likely to inject bacteria directly into their bloodstream through dirty needles. People with artificial valves are also at very high risk, especially during the first year after valve surgery. The risk is higher with an artificial aortic valve compared to a mitral valve and with a **mechanical valve** compared to an animal valve.

The source of infection in most affected individuals is infected gums; hence oral hygiene is very important.

Mechanical valve
An artificial valve with metallic components. These need to be anticoagulated.

45. What are the symptoms of infective endocarditis?

Acute bacterial endocarditis usually presents with a fever above 102°F, fast heart rate, fatigue, and extensive valve damage. The patients can also have symptoms related to valve damage, usually leakage, and can have severe sudden onset of shortness of breath.

Patients with sub acute bacterial endocarditis usually present with fatigue, milder fever (up to 101°F), weight loss, and low red blood cell count (anemia). These symptoms can last over a period of weeks to months before damage to the heart valves results in symptoms.

Arteries may become blocked if accumulations of bacteria and blood clots on the valves (called vegetations) break loose (becoming emboli), travel through the bloodstream to other parts of the body, and lodge in an artery, blocking it. Sometimes blockage can have serious consequences. Blockage of an artery to the brain can cause a stroke, and blockage of an artery to the heart can cause a heart attack. An **embolus** can also cause an infection in the area in which it lodges. Collections of pus (abscesses) may develop at the base of infected heart valves or wherever infected emboli settle.

Other symptoms may include chills, joint pain, paleness (**pallor**), painful nodules under the skin, and confusion. Small streaks of redness called splinter hemorrhages may appear under the fingernails. Tiny reddish spots may also appear on the skin and whites of the eyes. These spots and splinter hemorrhages are caused by small pieces (emboli) of the infected material (vegetation) from the infected valves. Larger emboli can cause stomach pain, blood in the urine, numbness in arms and legs, heart attack, stroke, new heart murmurs, or worsening of existing murmurs. The heart's electrical system may be affected, causing

Embolus

A solid particle that gets dislodged from one part of the circulation to another. Commonly, it is a thrombus (thromboembolism), less frequently an atheroma, piece of a tumor, vegetation, or air bubble.

Pallor

Pale skin color. This can occur because of anemia or low blood count.

the heart to slow down, which may cause sudden loss of consciousness or even death.

46. How is the diagnosis of infective endocarditis made?

Patients with infective endocarditis may have vague symptoms. Physicians can listen to the patients' hearts and detect murmurs. To help make the diagnosis, doctors usually perform echocardiography and obtain blood samples to test for the presence of bacteria. Usually, three or more blood samples are taken at different times on the same day. These blood tests (blood cultures) may identify the specific disease-causing bacteria and the best antibiotics to use against them. In people with heart abnormalities, doctors test their blood for bacteria before giving them antibiotics.

Echocardiography or ultrasound of the heart can show images of the heart valves and the infected masses on them (vegetations). Typically, transthoracic echocardiography (ultrasound probe placed on the chest wall) provides the diagnosis. It can show the vegetations, pockets of pus, valves involved, and abnormal leakage of blood through the valves, and it can detect the presence of tears in the valve leaflets. Sometimes, a transthoracic echocardiogram does not provide the information, and the patient may have to undergo a transesophageal echocardiogram (a procedure in which the ultrasound probe is passed down the throat into the esophagus or the food pipe just behind the heart). Transesophageal echocardiogram is more accurate and can detect smaller vegetations. It is also more invasive and costly.

47. Can infective endocarditis be prevented?

As a preventive measure, patients with artificial valves or congenital heart defects are given antibiotics before certain surgical, dental, and medical procedures. Consequently, surgeons, dentists, and other healthcare practitioners need to know if a person has had a heart valve disorder. Although the risk of endocarditis is not very high for these procedures and preventive antibiotics are not always effective, the consequences of endocarditis are so severe that most doctors believe that giving antibiotics before these procedures is a reasonable precaution.

48. How is endocarditis treated?

Once diagnosed with infective endocarditis, patients are treated with intravenous antibiotics for 4–8 weeks. In most cases, antibiotics alone may not be sufficient to cure a person, especially if an artificial valve is infected. Because antibiotics are given before heart valve replacement surgery to prevent infection, any bacteria that survive this treatment are probably resistant. Another reason is that it is generally harder to cure infection on artificial, implanted material than in human tissue.

Heart surgery may be needed to repair or replace damaged valves, remove vegetations, or drain abscesses (pockets of pus) if antibiotics do not work, a valve leaks severely, or a birth defect connects one chamber to another. Heart failure from significant valvular leaks can be fatal.

If untreated, infective endocarditis is always fatal. When treatment is given, risk of death depends on factors such as the person's age, duration of the infection, the presence of an artificial heart valve, and the type of infecting organism. Nonetheless, with aggressive antibiotic treatment, most people survive.

CONGENITAL VALVE PROBLEMS
49. What is a congenital lesion?

A congenital problem is one that is present from birth. The range of congenital cardiac abnormalities may range from a bicuspid aortic valve to complex valve problems to holes inside the heart to complex and multiple malformations.

50. What valves are affected?

A bicuspid aortic valve (where there are only two cusps instead of the normal three) is present in 2% of the population. This lesion is one form of acyanotic congenital valvular disease (there is no bluish discoloration of the lips or mucous membranes). Narrowing in the aortic valve area can also occur either below (subvalvular) or above (supravalvular) the valve. But these types of stenoses are rarer. A small number of patients with a bicuspid aortic valve can have narrowing of the aorta as well; this is called aortic coarctation. About 25% of patients with aortic coarctation have bicuspid aortic valves.

Ebstein's anomaly is another congenital valve lesion that involves the tricuspid valve. It is a rare disorder affecting about 1 in 200,000 live births. It accounts for less than 1% of all congenital lesions. This can be a form of cyanotic valve disease as there can be shunting of blood from the right to the left side (impure blood mixing with pure blood). The tricuspid valve is placed lower (more than 8 mm/m^2 of body surface area), compared to the mitral valve. An abnormal tricuspid valve leads to severe leakage.

Pulmonary stenosis

Narrowing of the pulmonary valve such that the right ventricle has to generate a higher pressure to pump blood into the lungs.

The pulmonary valve, which directs blood from the right ventricle to the pulmonary artery, can become narrowed. This is termed **pulmonary stenosis.** Subvalvular (below the valve) and supravalvular (above the valve) pulmonary stenosis can occur as well.

51. What are the symptoms?

Bicuspid aortic valve: Patients may not experience any symptoms until the valve is narrowed or becomes leaky. At advanced stages where the valve is too narrowed or leaky, patients may have shortness of breath, may not be able to lie flat in bed at night (orthopnea), and may develop frank heart failure.

Ebstein's anomaly: The classical symptoms of this valve disorder are cyanosis due to a right-to-left shunt, failure of the right ventricle, and palpitations due to arrhythmias (abnormal rhythms).

Pulmonary stenosis: Patients may complain of fatigue, shortness of breath, and abnormal rhythms.

52. How are these conditions diagnosed?

In the earlier stages of a bicuspid aortic valve, a physician can hear abnormal sounds called ejection click by a stethoscope. In advanced stages where there is narrowing or leakage, murmurs can be heard. When patients have heart failure, murmurs accompanied by abnormal lung sounds (called crackles) are heard.

Usually, in **Ebstein's anomaly** patients have signs of right heart failure. The jugular veins in the neck are engorged on examination. Murmurs can be heard by listening with a stethoscope, and patients have evidence of swelling in their feet.

Ebstein's anomaly

A congenital malformation of the tricuspid valve with apical displacement of one of its leaflets causing tricuspid regurgitation. This can be associated with arrhythmias as well.

A murmur can also be heard by stethoscope in those with pulmonary stenosis.

53. What diagnostic tests are useful in the diagnosis of these valve conditions?

Echocardiography: Echocardiography can be used to diagnose bicuspid aortic valve, Ebstein's anomaly, and pulmonary stenosis.

Echocardiography can detect the presence of a bicuspid aortic valve, as well as allow the physician to assess the severity of narrowing or leakage across the aortic valve. It can also help to assess the pressures inside the heart.

If Ebstein's anomaly is suspected, echocardiography can be used to detect the abnormally placed tricuspid valve, abnormal function of the right ventricle, leakage across the tricuspid valve (including its severity), the presence or absence of shunts, and pressures inside the heart.

Echocardiography can help in detecting the narrowing in the pulmonary valve, ascertaining the degree of narrowing, detecting pressure across the valve, and evaluating the function of the right ventricle.

Cardiac catheterization: This test can help detect abnormal pressures inside the left and right heart chambers.

Holter monitor: This monitor can be used to diagnose abnormal heart rate and rhythms.

PART THREE

Treatment Decisions

What needs to be done if there is a valve problem?

What are the general guidelines for surgical intervention?

Can you prevent valve problems?

More ...

54. What needs to be done if there is a valve problem?

If the valve problem is mild, generally no intervention is needed. If it is moderate, it is generally monitored unless there is a need for another heart surgery such as coronary artery bypass surgery, aortic surgery, or surgery for another valve. If the valve lesion is severe, then the need to intervene depends upon symptoms and the effect on heart function. If a severe valve problem is producing symptoms such as shortness of breath, chest pain, or exertional blackouts, then valve surgery may be warranted. A severe valve lesion may also impose an undue amount of workload on the heart. If there are signs of this, which is generally detectable by echocardiography, then valve surgery may be needed. The ultimate decision to operate or not depends upon a thorough risk/benefit analysis.

A severe valve lesion may also impose an undue amount of workload on the heart.

55. What are the general guidelines for surgical intervention?

Surgery is usually warranted for what can be broadly categorized as severe valve lesions producing symptoms and severe valve lesions producing damage to the heart, even without symptoms.

56. Can you prevent valve problems?

Most of the valve problems encountered in the United States are not preventable. The most common cause of aortic valve problem is a degenerative, calcific process that is age related and may be fuelled by the same risk factors as coronary artery disease, such as high choles-terol level, diabetes, high blood pressure, and kidney disease. The progression of this can potentially be retarded, but the efficacy of cholesterol lowering is yet to be convincingly established. In countries where rheumatic fever is still prevalent, it can be prevented by appropriate antibiotic treatment. Mitral valve prolapse is due to weakening of tissue, and there is no effective way of preventing its progression.

57. Who needs endocarditis prophylaxis?

Certain valve and congenital disorders of the heart are prone to infection if there are circulating bacteria in the blood after certain procedures. Taking antibiotics to prevent such infections is called endocarditis **pro-phylaxis**. *Endo* means inside, *card* means heart, and *itis* means infection or inflammation. Previously, the range of procedures and cardiac lesions for which prophylaxis was recommended were extensive. The current guide-lines are more restrictive. These are recommended only for oral procedures in patients with a **prosthetic valve**, in those with previous infections, and in patients with surgery for congenital heart surgery with residual lesions. Dentists have current recommendations and can offer the correct choice of antibiotic therapy. Notably, no prophylaxis is recommended for native valve lesions or mitral valve prolapse.

Prophylaxis
A measure used to prevent disease.

Prosthetic valve
Artificial valve made of tissue or metal.

PART FOUR

Surgical Management

What are the types of surgery for valve disorders?

What are the approaches for valve surgery?

What are the types of artificial valves?

More ...

58. What are the types of surgery for valve disorders?

An abnormally narrowed valve or a leaky valve in the aortic position is normally treated with valve replacement. Valve replacement is an open-heart surgery wherein the abnormal valve is removed and replaced with an artificial valve.

An abnormally narrowed mitral valve is usually treated with valve replacement with an artificial valve, through open-heart surgery. A leaky mitral valve due to myxomatous changes can be treated with repair of the valve, usually with resection of part of the leaflet, an **annuloplasty** ring, and sometimes adding artificial chordae tendinae. If the mitral valve is too floppy, then the valve might have to be replaced with an artificial valve, as repair may not be too durable. A leaky mitral valve due to abnormal enlargement of the left ventricle is usually treated with mitral valve repair with annuloplasty.

An abnormally narrowed tricuspid valve due to rheumatic causes is usually removed surgically and replaced with an artificial valve. Abnormal leakage of the tricuspid valve caused by dilatation of the annulus (functional cause) can be treated with repair of the tricuspid valve with annuloplasty.

An abnormally narrowed pulmonary valve can be treated with a balloon procedure called balloon **valvuloplasty**. A balloon is floated through the groin vein and positioned across the narrowed pulmonary valve and can be opened up under pressure, which enlarges

Annuloplasty

Surgical reduction in the size of the annulus to reduce or eliminate valvular regurgitation. Generally performed on mitral and tricuspid valves.

Valvuloplasty

Opening up a stenosed valve with a balloon, a device, or surgically.

the valve area. A leaky pulmonary valve is usually replaced with an artificial valve.

59. What are the approaches for valve surgery?

Valve surgery can involve either a **median sternotomy** or **minimally invasive** procedures.

In median sternotomy, the breastbone (sternum) is cut open, and, while the patient is on a heart and lung machine (cardiac bypass), the abnormal valve is visualized and replaced or repaired.

The mitral valve can be repaired through a smaller incision on the chest wall, which is a minimally invasive approach. The valve can also be repaired through robotic guidance using a minimally invasive approach. The minimally invasive and robotic approaches are technically more demanding and are available only in a few centers.

60. What are the types of artificial valves?

Artificial valves can be broadly divided into mechanical valves, bio-prosthetic valves. Xenograft, usually from pig or bovine origin, and **homograft**, obtained from human cadavers are forms of bio-prosthetic valves.

The earliest of the mechanical valves (Figure 9) used was the Starr-Edwards ball and cage valve. As the valve design became more technologically advanced,

Median sternotomy
A type of surgical procedure in which a vertical inline incision is made along the sternum, after which the sternum itself is divided, or "cracked."

Minimally invasive
A surgery performed without a large scar; it could be robotically assisted.

Homograft
Valve from a human cadaver used to replace a diseased valve in a patient.

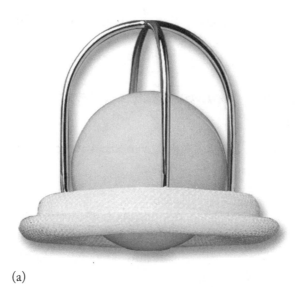

(a)

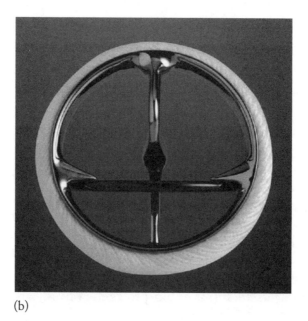

(b)

Figure 9 Mechanical valves: Broadly, the types include a caged ball valve such as Starr-Edward valve (not in use any more) [shown here], tilting disc valve such as Medtronic-Hall valve and Bileaflet valves such as St Jude and Carbomedics valves. The Bileaflet valves are being mostly used because of safety and favorable flow characteristics. ©Copyright Medtronic, Inc. Reprinted with permission. **(b) Mechanical valves: Medtronics-Hall.** ©Copyright Medtronic, Inc. Reprinted with permission.

newer models were introduced. Two of the newer types are the St. Jude bi leaflet mechanical valve and the Medtronic Hall mechanical valve.

Bioprosthetic valves (Figure 10) made from porcine or bovine origin are widely used; this is called a **xenograft**. Some of the newer valves are those made from the pericardial layer (lining covering the heart) from pigs.

In a homograft (Figure 11), valves harvested from human cadavers are utilized for valve replacement.

61. What are the major differences between mechanical and bioprosthetic valves?

Mechanical valves are metallic valves and are more durable. However, since this type of valve is metallic, it has a predisposition to form clots on the valve. If this type of valve is being used for valve replacement, long-term thinning of the blood (**anticoagulation**) with **warfarin** (**Coumadin**) is a must. Since the patients with mechanical valves are on warfarin, close follow-up is needed to accomplish adequate thinning of the blood.

Bioprosthetic valves like the xenograft and the homograft are made from biological tissues. Patients with these valves do not need blood thinning, but these valves are less durable than mechanical valves.

Treatment Decisions

Xenograft

An artificial or prosthetic valve made of animal tissue.

Anticoagulation

Process of thinning the blood using medication such as heparin or warfarin.

Warfarin

Blood thinner taken orally. It blocks the effect of vitamin K and works on the liver. This prevents blood clots on the mechanical valves and those in atrial fibrillation.

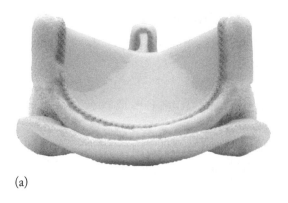

(a)

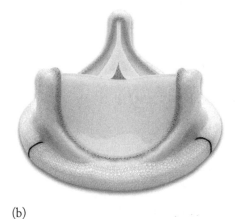

(b)

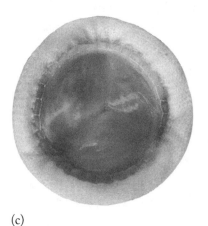

(c)

Figure 10   Bioprosthetic valves: These are tissue valves of bovine, porcine or pericardial ori-gin. Edwards Magna 3000 shown here. Image courtesy of Edwards Lifesciences, Irvine, California. **(b) Edwards Perimount mitral valve.** Image courtesy of Edwards Lifesciences, Irvine, California. **(c) Han-cock II aortic valve.** ©Copyright Medtronic, Inc. Reprinted with permission.

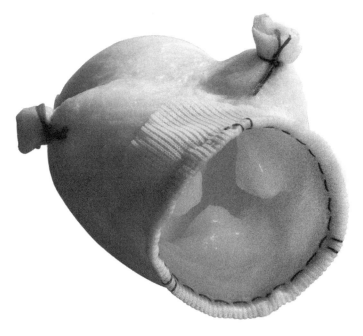

Figure 11   Homograft: This is a valve explanted from human cadavers.
©Copyright Medtronic, Inc. Reprinted with permission.

62. What are the risks and benefits of the different types of valves?

Though the mechanical valves are more durable and long lasting, these can be associated with some problems.

If the patient stops taking warfarin, the mechanical valve can get clotted, and the patient could get acute problems called valve thrombosis. Pieces of the clot can break off and cause blockage of an artery supplying the heart, arms and legs, or the brain (called an embolic phenomenon).

Patients who are on long-term warfarin therapy are at risk of their blood becoming thinned out too much. In that event, patients may have **bleeding** from the lining layers of the mouth and skin. The most dangerous type

Bleeding
Blood getting outside the blood vessels, generally because of damage to vessels or heart chambers.

51

of bleeding is bleeding in the brain, especially after trauma to the head from a fall, which can lead to stroke.

Mechanical valves are the valves of choice in young patients. Mechanical valves are a problem when they have to be used in a female patient of childbearing age. It poses a special problem, as these patients need warfarin therapy, which can cause birth defects when taken in the first trimester. If a patient of childbearing age has a mechanical valve and intends to become pregnant, a team approach involving a high-risk obstetrician, cardiologist, and the patient is needed. Such patients might need to be switched to therapy with heparin (to thin the blood) during the first trimester or for the entire duration of pregnancy. In this situation, a very close follow-up and monitoring are needed to keep the blood adequately thinned and to prevent the valve from clotting.

Bioprosthesis

An artificial valve made of animal or human tissue. It could be a porcine or bovine valve, a valve made of pericardium or a valve harvested from another human being postmortem. A human cadaveric derived valve is called a homograft.

Bioprosthetic valves last up to 10 years, less in younger individuals. **Bioprostheses** are more appropriate for patients over 70 years of age. These valves can form abnormal amounts of calcium deposits on them and can cause the valve to malfunction. This phenomenon is especially seen when the valves are implanted in younger individuals and in patients with kidney failure.

63. What are the long-term outcomes with artificial valves?

Mechanical valves last longer and the long-term outcomes with these valves are excellent.

Bioprosthetic valves usually do not last longer than 10 years. These valves either degenerate due to excess calcium deposition or can develop tears, at which time they need to be replaced.

Bioprosthetic valves usually do not last longer than 10 years.

64. How is the choice of valves made?

The choice for a particular type of valve for a given patient is made by the surgeon after discussion with the patient, taking into consideration his or her age, fall risk, bleeding risk, compliance, and whether the patient is a female of childbearing age. Patient preference is extremely important as well.

Mechanical valves are usually the choice of replacement in younger individuals as they are longer lasting and need warfarin therapy.

Bioprosthetic valves are the choices for patients aged 80 or older, younger patients with risks from warfarin therapy (this includes patients who are deemed noncompliant, and will not follow up for titration of warfarin), and females of childbearing age.

Treatment Decisions

65. What is anticoagulation? When is it used?

Anticoagulation is the process of artificially thinning the blood to prevent blood clotting inside the circulation. This can be performed using warfarin (old rat poison), heparin, or low molecular weight heparin. There are other less frequently used agents as well. Aspirin is an anti-platelet agent inhibiting the aggregation of platelets, which initiate clotting, or thrombosis. Hence, aspirin is not an **anticoagulant**, as it does not inhibit the blood proteins involved in the clotting process. Clopidogrel (Plavix) functions as a super-aspirin. To prevent clots on the artificial valves, inside the heart chambers, or the veins, anticoagulants are required.

Warfarin neutralizes the effects of vitamin K on the liver and reduces the production of clotting factors. Diet, antibiotics, liver disease, and several drugs modify its effects. Heparin and low molecular weight heparin are given by injection. Hence, warfarin is used for long-term therapy. It is generally indicated for mechanical valves, any clots inside the heart, and **atrial fibrillation**. In atrial fibrillation, the atrium does not contract, predisposing to atrial clots, which may cause stroke. This is common in valvular problems. Using warfarin, unless there is a contraindication such as bleeding, fall risk, or lack of compliance, reduces the stroke risk by about two thirds. Stroke is a devastating complication of atrial fibrillation.

Anticoagulant

Agent used to thin the blood.

Atrial fibrillation

A rhythm disorder in which the atria quiver instead of contracting. This can predispose to blood clots inside the atria and increase stroke risk and erratic heart rate response. It generally occurs because of enlarged atria, which can occur with valvular problems.

For artificial mechanical valves, the current recommendation is to use aspirin 81 mg per day in addition to warfarin.

66. What are the complications of warfarin therapy?

The main complication of warfarin is major bleeding such as bleeding into the brain causing stroke, or into the intestines or urinary tract. Patients should be very careful not to bump their head. Contact sports are proscribed. A bump on the head or a fall can result in subdural hematoma, which is bleeding inside the skull, but outside the brain. This can be life threatening and will need to be surgically drained. Hence, weakness on the sides or drowsiness in a patient on anticoagulation should arouse the suspicion of subdural hematoma. Many a times, the bump is very minor. Patients also need to be closely monitored for thinness of blood using a blood test measured by **international normalized ratio (INR)**. Normal INR is 1.0. Required thinness depends upon the reason for anticoagulation, and INR may vary from 1.8 to 3.5. INR is also affected by concomitant use of nonsteroidal drugs, antibiotics, vitamins, greens, and other drugs.

International normalized ratio (INR)

Method used to measure how thin the blood is and to adjust a dose of warfarin.

67. I have a mechanical valve, and I need surgery. What do I do with warfarin?

Ask your doctor before doing anything! Warfarin may need to be stopped before surgery unless it is a superficial surgery or minor oral surgery. The general recommendation is to bridge therapy with heparin (an intra-venous drug, with the dose adjusted based on blood tests) or enoxaparin (given subcutaneously twice a day, adjusted for body weight). This is begun when INR is sub therapeutic; it is stopped a few hours before surgery and started again as soon as possible after surgery and continued until INR is therapeutic after reinitiating warfarin therapy. The biggest danger of under anticoagulation is clotting of the mechanical valve, which is life threatening.

PART FIVE

Specific Valve Problems

What is mitral regurgitation?

What are the symptoms of mitral regurgitation?

What causes mitral regurgitation?

More ...

MITRAL REGURGITATION

68. What is mitral regurgitation?

Mitral regurgitation (Figure 4) is a leaky mitral valve. The mitral valve is a one-way valve, which allows blood to flow from the left atrium to the left ventricle and prevents it flowing back when the left ventricle contracts to pump blood (during systole) into the aorta. A mild amount of regurgitation is normal. When the leak is severe, it can increase the pressure in the left atrium and congest the lungs, resulting in shortness of breath. Stretching of the left atrium causes it to enlarge and may result in an irregular rhythm called atrial fibrillation. This can predispose a patient to stroke. As the left ventricle has to pump more blood, it may enlarge and also weaken.

69. What are the symptoms of mitral regurgitation?

In severe lesions, one may get shortness of breath at rest or with exertion. One may also get tired or feel palpitations. Atrial fibrillation can cause stroke or blood clots in the limbs. Many of the patients with severe mitral regurgitation have no symptoms because the heart has compensated or the patient has learned to live with lesser degrees of activity. This phenomenon is common in patients with valvular diseases, because the progression is slow, hence patients deny symptoms despite significant impairment. Symptoms dictate if surgery is needed; hence patients should think carefully, considering their efforts at climbing stairs, etc., before telling their doctor they have no symptoms. One's doctor can objectively assess exercise capacity by doing a formal exercise stress test that involves the patient walking on a treadmill or using a bicycle ergometer.

Dr. SP comments:

It is important to remember that the symptoms may be very subtle even with severe disease, and you may question the need for surgery. Have your doctor review your echocardiogram with you to understand the severity of regurgitation. Sometimes, a picture is worth a thousand words!

70. What causes mitral regurgitation?

Mitral regurgitation occurs when the two mitral leaflets cannot close well, leaving a "hole" in the valve. This can occur because of damage to the valve leaflets by processes such as endocarditis or rheumatic fever. Sometimes leaflets may be intact, but one or both of them may either bend excessively into the left atrium (prolapse) or may be prevented from coming to the coaptation plane. This occurs when the left ventricle is excessively dilated in **cardiomyopathy** or deformed as after a heart attack. The latter entity is called ischemic mitral regurgitation.

Cardiomyopathy

Heart muscle disease. Broadly, there are four types: dilated, hypertrophic, restrictive, and obliterative.

71. What treatment options are available for severe mitral regurgitation?

Generally, timing of intervention depends upon three things—whether there are symptoms, if there is damage to the left ventricle, and if the valve can be repaired without a need for replacement. Generally, asymptomatic patients with normal heart size and function are closely followed. If there are symptoms such as shortness of breath, then valve surgery may be needed. The type of valve surgery would depend upon the valve anatomy and age. If the valve is repairable and expertise is available, then repair should be done. Eighty percent of the valves should be repairable in the hands of a competent surgeon (Figure 12). Mitral valve repair is specialized and preferable to replacement; it is preferable to discuss with your surgeon his and his institution's repair volume. Repair needs a team of a cardiothoracic surgeon, a cardiologist, and an anesthesiologist. If the valve is not repairable, then replacement is performed. In young individuals, a mechanical valve is preferred as it is more durable. In older individuals, tissue valves are recommended. Percutaneous or catheter-based technologies are still experimental, their durability is not known, and the techniques are still in evolution.

In older individuals, tissue valves are recommended.

72. What about minimally invasive surgery?

Conventional surgery includes a complete sternotomy, which means completely cutting open the breastbone to expose the heart, and the patient should have a cardiopulmonary bypass to stop the heart temporarily. In less invasive approaches, only the upper breastbone is split open or an incision may be placed on the right side of the chest. The other technique is robotically assisted surgery, in which four smaller incisions are

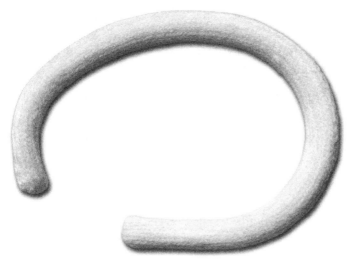

(a)

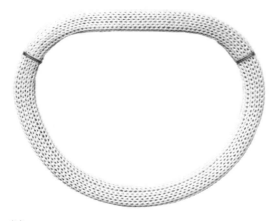

(b)

Figure 12   Mitral annuloplasty rings which are used to narrow the mitral orifice to facilitate co-aptation of the leaflets to eliminate mitral regurgitation. Other techniques include resection of part of the leaflet and insertion of artificial chords to repair mitral regurgitation.

made and surgery is performed by robotic arms controlled by the surgeon using a computer. These need special training, expertise, and comfort level, and not all surgeons prefer it for various reasons. Very few centers in the United States have a high-volume of robotically assisted valve surgery program. Some of the most well-known centers do not prefer robotically assisted surgery and are proponents of traditional approaches with which they may have outstanding results.

Dr. SP comments:

It is extremely important to be proactive and to research the centers for surgical repair or replacement of your heart valve. Most large institutions have web-based information that is easily accessible, as are their success rates for different types of procedures. Ask your cardiologist where he/she would go to have the valve surgery himself or herself if they needed it. You should feel pretty comfortable going to the same place provided other issues such as traveling, lodging, and medical insurance are covered. If you cannot or do not have the financial resources to go to the best hospital, research the experience of all available local hospitals prior to making your choice.

73. Are there nonsurgical approaches available for severe mitral regurgitation?

There are some catheter-based approaches under investigation. These are available strictly under research protocols to study if they are durable and useful. The catheter is passed to the valve through the groin to deliver therapy. One of the experimental devices is a clip that pinches the two mitral leaflets together. In another approach, a ring is placed around the mitral annulus through the coronary sinus to tighten the valve. There are multiple device companies working on these innovations, and the verdict on their efficacy in selected subsets of patients should be available in a few years. In patients with severe functional mitral regurgitation with a dilated, poorly functioning left ventricle, such as that seen in heart failure settings, aggressive antifailure therapy with **angiotensin converting enzyme inhibitors** (ACE inhibitors) and **beta-blockers** frequently may improve the heart size and function and eliminate mitral regurgitation. A similar phenomenon may also be seen with a special pacemaker called a biventricular pacemaker, which is frequently used in patients with severe heart failure.

74. I have mitral valve prolapse with severe regurgitation, but no symptoms. Should I have surgery?

This area is hotly debated. Regurgitation is not going to go away; it can cause ventricular damage and result in atrial fibrillation. Hence, after a thorough evaluation with echocardiography, if there is a good chance that the valve can be repaired without replacement and surgical expertise exists to repair it, then repair is not unreasonable. It should, however, be pointed out that the higher the repair volume in an institution, the higher the repair success and durability rates.

Angiotensin converting enzyme inhibitor

A type of medication that blocks the effect of angiotensin II and dilates the blood vessels. It lowers blood pressure.

Beta-blocker

A medication that blocks the beta receptor, which is a receptor for adrenaline and noradrenaline. The beta-blockers slow the heart rate and lower the blood pressure. They are also protective in patients with heart attacks and heart failure.

75. What are the determinants of mitral valve repair success?

The success of mitral valve repair depends upon the cause of regurgitation, the extent of valvular abnormality, the experience of the surgeon, the experience of the cardiologist, and the use of artificial chords. Localized flail or limited prolapse of the posterior leaflet is more easily repaired than a diffusely prolapsing valve. Posterior leaflet is easier to repair than the anterior leaflet. Ischemic and rheumatic valves are more difficult to repair and less durable. High-volume institutions have a better outcome, hence one should ask about annual repair volume and what percentages of valves are repaired. In good centers, 80% of valves are repaired, as repair is better than replacement. There is data to indicate that use of artificial chords increases repair durability. Annuloplasty is used in all repairs.

Dr. SP comments:

Preoperative preparation, both medical and emotional, is a must. Following your cardiologist's orders and taking all prescribed medications gets you into optimal shape for surgery and helps shorten your recovery time. Many large surgical centers offer programs to allay anxiety with relaxation techniques such as taped music and creative visualizations. There usually are consultations with all team members, including the cardiologist, the cardiovascular surgeon, and the cardiac anesthesiologist. This is the time to ask any questions that you may have and [the time to make sure you] have a clear understanding of the process from the presurgical preparation to the discharge from the hospital. Also, don't worry if you are asked the same questions by many different personnel on the day of your surgery. These are called identifiers and are safety features that hospitals use to make sure that the correct procedure is being done on the correct patient by the correct surgeon.

Pain management is used postoperatively. But after the third postoperative day, you should feel well enough to use pain medication only occasionally.

Cardiac rehabilitation starts during your hospital stay and usually lasts 3 to 4 months depending on your heart condition. Faithful attendance at all your appointments greatly facilitates your recovery. Rehab professionals watch your progress and encourage you to reach your full exercise potential.

MITRAL STENOSIS
76. What is mitral stenosis, and what are the causes?

Mitral stenosis refers to narrowing of the mitral valve such that there is obstruction or resistance for blood to flow from the left atrium to the left ventricle. The normal opening of the mitral valve is about 5 cm^2. When the area drops to 1 cm^2, the stenosis is severe. When stenosis occurs, the pressure in the left atrium increases, which causes the blood to back up in the lungs, and the blood pressure in the lungs increases. This causes shortness of breath and may also cause atrial fibrillation. The most common cause of mitral stenosis worldwide is rheumatic fever. In rheumatic fever, inflammation in the valve leaflets leads to adhesion, deposition of fibrous tissue, and calcium, resulting in valve narrowing. With the aging population, calcific or degenerative stenosis is becoming frequent as well. In this process, calcium gets deposited at the periphery of the valve leaflets, ultimately encroaching onto the leaflet body, making it stiffer and impeding valve opening. There are congenital causes as well.

77. What are the symptoms of mitral stenosis?

Milder degrees of mitral stenosis are asymptomatic. In severe cases, shortness of breath is the principal symptom and occurs on exertion. Palpitations can occur when atrial fibrillation develops. Shortness of breath will increase as well with atrial fibrillation. Stroke as a presenting symptom is not uncommon and is more common in older patients who go into atrial fibrillation. Rarely, patients can cough up blood as well due to rupture of bronchial blood vessels caused by high pressure inside the lungs. Fatigue is common due to reduced cardiac output by the heart. Dizzy spells and chest pain are uncommon.

78. How is mitral stenosis diagnosed and evaluated?

Physical examination may reveal the typical murmur and opening snap of the valve and features of high pulmonary artery pressure. Diagnosis is established by echocardiography. This helps assess stenosis severity, amount of regurgitation, and valve morphology, which is important in deciding if the valve is suitable for balloon valvuloplasty. Generally, significant regurgitation, severe calcification, and thickening of the valve or excessive thickening and matting of the chordae tendinae make percutaneous valvuloplasty less desirable.

79. What are the treatment options in mitral stenosis?

Slowing the heart rate with a beta-blocker is useful as it gives more time for the left atrium to empty. If there is atrial fibrillation, patients should be on a blood thinner such as warfarin to prevent a blood clot and stroke. In symptomatic patients with severe stenosis, two options are percutaneous valvuloplasty and valve replacement. Percutaneous valvuloplasty is feasible when valve appearance on echocardiography is conducive to valvotomy and there is not much of mitral regurgitation. In other instances, especially when an additional cardiac reparative surgery is needed, valve replacement is indicated.

AORTIC STENOSIS
80. What is aortic stenosis?

Aortic stenosis is narrowing of the aortic valve causing obstruction to blood flow. Generally, this occurs at the level of the valve, though processes below or above the valve can cause stenosis as well, although this rarely occurs. Stenosis is graded mild to severe based on the aortic valve area or how much the valve opens. Normal opening in an adult is about 3.0 cm^2. Severe aortic stenosis is deemed to exist if the valve area is less than 1

Aortic stenosis

Narrowing of the aortic valve such that the left ventricle has to generate a higher pressure to pump blood.

cm^2. In the presence of aortic stenosis, the left ventricle has to work harder and has to generate a higher pressure to pump blood across the stenosed valve. Because of this, the left ventricular wall becomes thicker (hypertrophy). If the severe stenosis is unrelieved for a long time, the left ventricle can ultimately fail.

81. What causes aortic stenosis?

Generally, valvular aortic stenosis is due to calcium deposition—this is called calcific or degenerative aortic stenosis. This process is similar to atherosclerosis and hence is found in individuals older than 70 years of age. In younger individuals, aortic stenosis is more likely due to a bicuspid valve, a situation where there are two leaflets instead of three. This is present in about 2% of the population, but only a small fraction of these individuals develop aortic stenosis or regurgitation.

82. What are the symptoms of aortic stenosis?

Once symptoms develop, risk to life increases if stenosis is uncorrected.

Even with severe aortic stenosis, many individuals are asymptomatic, and some learn to live with symptoms and cut down on activities and deny symptoms when asked. Symptoms are important to ascertain in order to decide if the patient needs aortic valve replacement. Once symptoms develop, risk to life increases if stenosis is uncorrected. The cardinal symptoms of aortic stenosis are exertional shortness of breath, chest pain, or blackouts. These are exertional because a narrowed valve does not allow an increase in output from the heart, which is needed during exertion as muscles need higher blood supply.

Many of the patients with severe aortic stenosis have no symptoms because the heart has compensated or the patient has learned to live with lesser degrees of activity. This phenomenon is common in patients with valvular diseases as the progression is slow, hence patients deny symptoms despite significant impairment. Symptoms dictate if surgery is needed; hence patients should think carefully, considering their efforts at climbing stairs, etc., before telling their doctor they have no symptoms. One's doctor can objectively assess exercise capacity by doing a formal exercise stress test that involves the patient walking on a treadmill or using a bicycle ergometer. About 50% of patients with severe aortic stenosis who are truly symptomatic initially deny symptoms and develop symptoms for the first time when they get on the treadmill! Humans are very versatile and adapt rapidly to physical limitations!

83. When do you replace the aortic valve?

General indications for valve replacement include symptomatic severe aortic stenosis, or stenosis causing weakening of the heart muscle or need for another heart surgery, though the valve is not producing symptoms or is only moderately severe. With the tissue valves becoming more durable and surgical risk becoming less, the threshold for surgery may go down in the future. There are investigational valves that can be deployed over catheters similar to a stent without opening the chest.

84. I am 82 years old, have severe aortic stenosis, and I am told my heart muscle is weak. Am I still a candidate for surgery?

Absolutely, unless there is some other contraindication. Age is not a contraindication. Aortic stenosis is the disease of the elderly. Even the presence of severe weakening of the heart muscle is not a contraindication as long as aortic stenosis is severe. Replacing the valve is likely to improve the ventricular function as the ventricle can pump more easily. Severe pulmonary hypertension is not a contraindication either. In all these groups, there is a huge survival advantage with valve replacement, and valve replacement can be performed with reasonable mortality and morbidity. In these patients, outcome without valve surgery is dismal. Having said this, there is a huge under treatment of these patients, mostly due to hesitation on the part of the physicians to recommend surgery.

In aortic stenosis and mitral regurgitation, it is common for patients to downplay symptoms. After surgery most of them are able to do a lot more and will say they never felt better and enjoy the markedly improved physical capacity.

85. What is patient-prosthesis mismatch?

When the valve size is too small for the body size, the situation is referred to as patient-prosthesis mismatch. Body size is a rough guide to valve size needs. Body size is measured in terms of body surface area, which is obtained from weight and height. Normal body surface area is about 1.8 m^2. Valve size is measured in terms of effective valve area. For a prosthetic aortic valve, an effective valve area greater than 0.85 cm^2/m^2 is ideal and patient-prosthesis mismatch is deemed to exist when it is less than 0.65 cm^2/m^2. To prevent patient-prosthesis mismatch, the surgeon would put in the biggest valve that can be fitted during surgery. For the aortic position, a valve size 23 mm or greater is generally adequate. If the area is small, sometimes the surgeon can enlarge the area before suturing the valve.

86. Am I a candidate for percutaneous valve therapy?

Several percutaneous valve models are in clinical trials. This type of valve can be delivered without taking the old one out, over a catheter-based system (Figure 13). The technology is feasible, and pulmonary and aortic valves have been replaced with this technology. Its safety, clinical benefit, and long-term durability are being investigated. Generally, these trials are enrolling very high-surgical-risk patients and patients who have been turned down for surgery. The Food and Drug Administration has not yet approved percutaneous

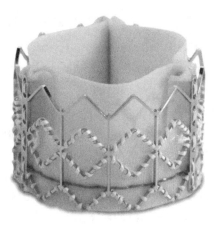

Figure 13 Percutaneous aortic valve: An example of an aortic valve which can be implanted without open heart surgery. These are still in trials in high risk patients who are not ideal or non candidates for surgical valve replacement.

valve therapy for common use. The technology looks very promising, especially in high-risk patients.

AORTIC REGURGITATION
87. What is aortic regurgitation?

Aortic regurgitation is a leaky aortic valve such that blood leaks back from the aorta into the left ventricle during **diastole**. Diastole is the period during which the left ventricle is relaxing and receiving blood from the left atrium and blood in the aorta flows forward. An aortic valve is a unidirectional valve designed to allow blood to flow from the left ventricle into the aorta, but not in the opposite direction. Aortic regurgitation can be anywhere from mild to severe and causes

Diastole

Phase of the cardiac cycle during which the ventricles are not contracting. The ventricles fill with blood during this period.

the left ventricle to overfill and work harder. Because of this, patients can develop shortness of breath, fatigue, and heart failure. It can also be acute, which means occurring suddenly, and it may be due to infection of the valve (endocarditis) or a tear in the ascending aorta extending into the valve (**aortic dissection**). Acute aortic regurgitation is life threatening and is a surgical emergency. Chronic regurgitation has an insidious onset and is slowly progressive due to a variety of causes such as valve degeneration, rheumatic fever, a bicuspid valve, or aortic dilation.

88. What symptoms does aortic regurgitation produce, and how is it diagnosed?

Aortic regurgitation might have no symptoms, or it can have very severe symptoms. Shortness of breath on exertion and fatigue are principal symptoms. In chronic aortic regurgitation, the symptoms are insidious and can be unappreciated by the patient. Clinically, the diagnosis can be made by the characteristic diastolic murmur that can be heard with the stethoscope, as well as by several peripheral signs, including bobbing of the head. The diagnosis is made by echocardiography, which can quantitate the amount of regurgitation, reason for regurgitation, heart function, and pulmonary artery pressure. Cardiac catheterization is generally performed in preparation for surgery in those older than 35 years to rule out blockages to the

Aortic dissection
A tear in the wall of the aorta, which may be life threatening, due to aortic rupture. Common causes are hypertension, Marfan syndrome, and conditions causing weakening of arterial wall.

Specific Valve Problems

coronary arteries, which can be fixed at the same time as aortic valve replacement.

89. What is the treatment for aortic regurgitation?

Symptomatic severe aortic regurgitation and acute severe regurgitation warrant aortic valve replacement. Lesser degrees of regurgitation are monitored, and underlying causes, if any, are treated (e.g., rheumatic fever, endocarditis). If the regurgitation is due to **aortic root** dilation, good blood pressure control is important. The decision for surgery in such patients depends upon the severity of regurgitation, ventricular size and function, and aortic size. If the aorta is severely dilated, it would need to be replaced as well to prevent rupture, which could be instantaneously lethal. If the regurgitation is severe but not producing symptoms, there may be a role for medications such as nifedipine.

Aortic root

Part of the ascending aorta immediately above the aortic valve.

90. What is aortic dissection, and how can it involve an aortic valve?

Aortic dissection refers to a tear in the wall of the aorta; it can be life threatening as it may cause rupture of the aorta into the chest or the pericardium. Acute dissection is a medical and potentially a surgical emergency. Dissection involving the ascending aorta is more dangerous as it may rupture into the pericardium, obstruct the coronary arteries, or tear into the aortic valve, causing it to leak. Involvement of the aortic valve will cause regurgitation. Ascending aortic dissection is a surgical emergency needing emergent surgery by an experienced surgeon. The door-to-operating room time has to be as short as possible as mortality is 1–2% per hour. Patients should not be sent for angiography before surgery as it delays surgery, is not needed, and increases the risk of renal failure.

91. What is Marfan syndrome, and does it affect the valves?

Marfan syndrome is a genetically mediated connective tissue disease caused by abnormal collagen, which weakens the aortic wall and the valves. It is an autosomal dominant disease; hence first-degree relatives of those with the syndrome may be affected as well. Weakening of the aortic wall can cause dilatation of the aorta (aneurysm), which runs the risk of rupture or dissection. This risk can be reduced by beta-blocker therapy. When the aortic diameter is 4.5–5.0 cm, it may need to be surgically replaced. Aortic dilation or dissection can cause aortic regurgitation. Weak supporting structures (chordae tendinae) of the mitral valve can cause mitral valve prolapse and regurgitation.

Marfan syndrome

A genetic disorder causing weakening of connective tissue. Features include tall stature, dislocation of ocular lens, valve prolapse, and aortic aneurysm.

92. What is a Ross procedure?

A **Ross procedure** is a technique for aortic valve replacement first performed by Dr. Ross in London, England. In this procedure, the patient's own pulmonary valve is excised to replace the aortic valve. The pulmonary valve is replaced by a homograft, which is a cadaveric valve. The rationale for this procedure is that

Ross procedure

A surgical procedure in which a patient's own pulmonary valve is used to replace the aortic valve and a homograft is used to replace the explanted pulmonary valve.

Autograft

A valve from one's own body. For example, in a Ross procedure, a patient's own pulmonary valve (autograft) is used to replace a diseased aortic valve. The excised pulmonary valve is replaced by a homograft.

the pulmonary **autograft** is a living tissue and will grow with the body; hence is generally performed in children. The surgery is extensive and demanding. Also, a single valve problem is converted into a two-valve problem. The advantage of this procedure is that no anticoagulation is required and the neoaortic valve grows. The problems could be neoaortic valve regurgitation, neoaortic root dilatation, and late stenosis of pulmonary homograft.

TRICUSPID VALVE DISEASE

93. What is the importance of tricuspid regurgitation?

The tricuspid valve was until now considered an orphan valve and its regurgitation was not deemed to be important. But now we know that its regurgitation can cause problems when severe. It can cause fatigue and can adversely affect the function of the right ventricle, which bears the brunt of the leak. Most of the surgical interventions on the tricuspid valve are in conjunction with some other important valve surgery, but primary repair is becoming more common. The preferred surgical procedure is repair. Bio-prosthetic valves in this location are not very durable, and mechanical valves clot very easily despite adequate thinning of the blood with warfarin.

94. I have severe tricuspid regurgitation, and I am told my pulmonary artery pressure is very high

(severe pulmonary hypertension). Will surgery for tricuspid valve help?

Surgery will not help unless you have another problem that is causing your severe pulmonary hypertension, which can also be addressed at the same time and would result in lowering your pulmonary pressure. An example of this is mitral valve disease. This can occasionally cause severe pulmonary hypertension, which can be reversed by mitral valve repair or replacement. The reason for tricuspid regurgitation in your case could be high pulmonary artery pressure, which can cause dilation of the right ventricle and tricuspid annulus, thus causing tricuspid regurgitation. This generally regresses with lowering of pulmonary pressure. This type of regurgitation is called functional tricuspid regurgitation. If surgery is being performed for other valves, then tricuspid annuloplasty is warranted as well. Tricuspid regurgitation will not cause pulmonary hypertension. Normal pulmonary artery systolic pressure is about 25 mm Hg (for comparison, systolic blood pressure in the aorta, which is measured by a blood pressure cuff, is about 120 mm Hg). Severe pulmonary hypertension exists when it exceeds about 70 mm Hg.

95. What is a flail tricuspid valve?

Flail valve is a valve that has lost support because of a ruptured chordae tendinae. Tricuspid valve has three leaflets supported by chordae tendinae coming from three papillary muscles attached to the right ventricular walls. When one of these chordae snaps, the corresponding valve leaflet will become flail and prolapses

Flail valve

Loss of support to the valve, generally due to torn chordae tendinae, causing valvular regurgitation. It can affect the mitral or tricuspid valve.

abnormally into the right atrium due to loss of support. This will result in tricuspid regurgitation, which could be severe. The common reasons for flail tricuspid valve include blunt chest trauma, as in a motor vehicle accident with pressure from the steering wheel, and rarely after heart biopsy using a catheter (endomyocardial biopsy). Mostly, these are asymptomatic and unrecognized. When there is severe tricuspid regurgitation, fatigue may develop and the right ventricle may weaken due to volume overload. Under these circumstances, tricuspid valve repair is indicated.

96. What is tricuspid stenosis?

Tricuspid stenosis

Narrowing of the tricuspid valve such that the right atrial pressure rises to push blood across the stenosed valve.

Carcinoid syndrome

A hormone-secreting tumor manifesting with flushing, diarrhea, and valvular problems mostly affecting the right side of the heart.

Tricuspid stenosis refers to narrowing of the tricuspid valve producing obstruction to blood flow from the right atrium to the right ventricle. It is very rare and may be due to rheumatic heart disease or **carcinoid syndrome** (a tumor producing some chemicals such as serotonin, which causes inflammation and thickening of the valve). When severe, this is generally amenable to balloon valvuloplasty. The other cause of tricuspid stenosis is malfunctioning prosthetic valve. A bioprosthetic valve in tricuspid position has a propensity to undergo degeneration and can rapidly stenose. Mechanical valves in this position are very predisposed to thrombosis and obstruction.

PULMONARY VALVE DISEASE
97. What is pulmonary stenosis?

Pulmonary stenosis (PS) refers to narrowing of the pulmonary valve or the area just below or above the valve. The most common reason it occurs is due to congenital malformation, but it rarely can occur due to carcinoid syndrome or rheumatic fever. The narrowing would require the right ventricle to generate a higher pressure to be able to pump blood across the narrowed valve. As a consequence, the right ventricle becomes thicker and may fail. In severe cases, the right ventricle generates a pressure equal to or greater than the left ventricle (normally right ventricular pressure is about one sixth the left ventricular pressure). The symptoms may include fatigue, chest pain, shortness of breath, or exertional dizziness. PS is better tolerated than aortic stenosis. Most of the valvular cases of severe PS are amenable to balloon valvuloplasty. When it is not, surgery is indicated.

98. Is pulmonary regurgitation important?

Small amounts of regurgitation are normal at the pulmonary valve. Severe degrees may impose an extra load on the right ventricle, which may dilate and eventually fail. Tricuspid and **pulmonary regurgitations** were formerly largely neglected. But it is being increasingly recognized that these are important lesions that may lead to morbidity and mortality. If pulmonary regurgitation is severe and causing symptoms such as reduced exercise tolerance or causing right ventricular dysfunction (weakening), then valve replacement may be warranted. Traditionally, a bioprosthetic valve such as a homograft is implanted surgically. But percutaneous valves (implanted using a catheter without opening the

Pulmonary regurgitation

Leaky pulmonary valve such that blood leaks back from the pulmonary artery into the right ventricle.

chest) are being tried in research studies and seem to be promising.

99. I had repair of tetralogy of Fallot in childhood. Recently, I have been told there is severe pulmonary regurgitation. Do I need surgery?

Tetralogy of Fallot

A congenital cyanotic (blue skin color because of low oxygen content) heart disease consisting of pulmonary stenosis, large ventricular septal defect, right ventricular hypertrophy, and aorta overriding the ventricular septal defect.

Babies with this condition are born blue because of lack of adequate oxygen in their blood.

Tetralogy of Fallot is a congenital heart disease with ventricular septal defect (a hole in the wall between two ventricles), aorta overriding this defect, right ventricular hypertrophy, and pulmonary stenosis. Babies with this condition are born blue because of lack of adequate oxygen in their blood. The repair includes closing the ventricular septal defect and relieving pulmonary stenosis. Sometimes, surgery on the malformed pulmonary valve could be complex, leading to pulmonary regurgitation, which may progress. One of the risks of this is progressive dilation and weakening of the right ventricle. Some patients have a thick, noncompliant right ventricle, which may cause severe right-sided heart failure, liver congestion, and swelling in the legs.

The decision to replace a pulmonary valve depends upon the degree of regurgitation (it has to be severe), presence of symptoms such as fatigue/shortness of breath, presence of heart failure, and presence of right ventricular dysfunction. Pulmonary valve replacement is the treatment, if needed. Percutaneous pulmonary valve replacement may be available in the future.

100. Where can I find more details on valvular problems?

The following are useful resources:

The American Heart Association website topic on how the heart works: *http://www.americanheart.org/presenter.jhtml?identifier=1557#*

and

http://www.americanheart.org/presenter.jhtml?identifier=4642

The American Heart Association website also includes various heart-related topics available at: *http://www.americanheart.org/presenter.jhtml?identifier=555*

Bonow RO, Carabello BA, Chatterjee K, de Leon AC Jr, Faxon DP, Freed MD, et al. ACC/AHA 2006 guidelines on management of valvular heart disease: a report of the American College of Cardiology/American Heart Association task force on practice guidelines. 2006. Available at: *http://www.americanheart.org/downloadable/heart/1150461625693Valvular HeartDisease2006.pdf*

Hirsch J, Fuster V, Ansell J, Halperin JL. American Heart Association/American College of Cardiology Foundation guide to warfarin therapy. Circulation. 2003;107:1692-1711. Available at: *http://circ.ahajournals.org/cgi/reprint/107/12/1692*

Wilson W, Taubert K, Gewitz M, Lockhart P, Baddour L, Levison M, et al. B) American Heart Association guidelines on prevention of infective endocarditis: guidelines from the American Heart Association. 2007. Available at: *http://circ.ahajournals.org/cgi/reprint/CIRCULATIONAHA.106.183095*

Recent Key Publications From The Authors Related to Valvular Issues

Aortic Valves

Kapoor N, Varadarajan P, Pai RG. Echocardiographic predictors of pulmonary hypertension in patients with severe aortic stenosis. *Eur J Echocardiogr.* March 16, 2007:84:85–86

Pai RG. Degenerative valve disease [letter]. *J Am Coll Cardiol.* December 2006;19;48(12):2601.

Pai RG. Statins and aortic stenosis progression: are biologic targets still an option? *Curr Cardiol Reports.* November 2005;7(6):399–400.

Pai RG, Varadarajan P. Aortic valve replacement in asymptomatic aortic stenosis: time to reconsider "watchful expectancy." *Ann Thorac Surg.* 2007;84:356–357.

Pai RG, Varadarajan P, Kapoor N, Bansal RC. Aortic valve replacement improves survival in severe aortic stenosis associated with severe pulmonary hypertension. *Ann Thorac Surg.* July 2007;84(1):80–85.

Pai RG, Varadarajan P, Kapoor N, Bansal RC. Malignant Natural History of Asymptomatic Severe Aortic Stenosis: Benefit of Aortic Valve Replacement. *Annals Thoracic Surg.* 2006;82:2116–2122.

Palta S, Gill KS, Pai RG. Role of inadequate adaptive LV hypertrophy in the genesis of mitral regurgitation in patients with severe aortic stenosis: implications for its prevention. *J Heart Valve Dis.* 2003;12:601–604.

Palta S, Pai AM, Gill KS, Pai RG. New insights into the progression of aortic stenosis: implications for secondary prevention. *Circulation.* 2000;101:2497–2502.

Varadarajan P, Kapoor N, Bansal RC, Pai RG. Clinical profile and natural history of 453 nonsurgically managed patients with severe aortic stenosis. *Ann Thorac Surg.* 2006;82:2111–2115.

Varadarajan P, Kapoor N, Bansal RC, Pai RG. Survival in elderly patients with severe aortic stenosis is dramatically improved by aortic valve replacement: results from a cohort of 277 patients aged >/=80 years. *Eur J Cardiothorac Surg.* November 2006;30(5):722–727.

Mitral Valve

Campwala SZ, Bansal RC, Wang N, Razzouk A, Pai RG. Factors affecting regression of mitral regurgitation following isolated coronary artery bypass surgery. *Eur J Cardiothorac Surg.* 2005 Nov;28(5):783–787.

Campwala SZ, Bansal RC, Wang N, Razzouk A, Pai RG. Mitral regurgitation progression following isolated coronary artery bypass surgery: frequency, risk factors, and potential prevention strategies. *Eur J Cardiothorac Surg.* 2006 Mar;29(3):348–353. [Epub 2006 Jan 24).

Pai RG. Echocardiographic assessment of myocardial viability. *ACC Educational Highlights.* 1995;11:1-5.

Pai RG, Jintapakorn W, Tanimoto M, Cao Q, Pandian N, Shah PM. Three-dimensional echocardiographic reconstruction of left ventricular volume by a trans-esophageal tomographic technique: in vitro and in vivo validation of its volume. *Echocardiography.* 1996;13:613–621.

Pai RG, Jintapakorn W, Tanimoto M, Shah PM. Role for Papillary Muscle Position and Mitral Valve Structure in Systolic Anterior Motion of the Mitral Leaflets in Hyperdynamic Left Ventricular Function. *Am J Cardiol.* 1995;76:623–628.

Pai RG, Shah PM. Functional significance of a flexible mitral annuloplasty ring: a three-dimensional echocardiographic assessment [editorial]. *J Heart Valve Dis.* 1995;4:615–617.

Pai RG, Tanimoto M, Jintapakorn W, Azevedo J, Pandian N, Shah PM. Dynamic three-dimensional anatomy of the mitral annulus by transesophageal echo-CT technique. *J Heart Valve Dis.* 1995;4:623–627.

Pai RG, Varadarajan P, Tanimoto M. Effect of atrial fibrillation on the dynamics of mitral annular area. *J Heart Valve Dis.* 2003;12:31–37.

Tanimoto M, Pai RG. Effect of left atrial enlargement on mitral annular size: its role in the genesis of mitral regurgitation in patients with structurally normal mitral leaflets. *Am J Cardiol.* 1996;77:769–774.

Varadarajan P, Sharma S, Heywood JT, Pai RG. High prevalence of clinically silent severe mitral regurgitation in heart failure patients: role for echocardiography. *J Am Soc Echocardiogr.* 2006;19:1458–1461.

Wang N, Campwala S, Habibipour S, Hodgins D, Pai R, Razzouk A. Impact of mitral insufficiency on reoperative coronary artery surgery in ischemic cardiomyopathy patients. *Eur J Cardiothorac Surg.* 2004;26:1118–1128.

Specific Valve Problems

Glossary

Abscess: Collection of pus due to bacterial infection.

Aneurysm: Abnormal dilatation of an artery or a cardiac chamber. A dilated blood vessel increases the risk of rupture.

Angina: Chest pain due to lack of blood supply to the heart muscle. This generally occurs due to a blockage in the coronary artery. Generally, the chest pain is exertional.

Angiotensin converting enzyme inhibitor: A type of medication that blocks the effect of angiotensin II and dilates the blood vessels. It lowers blood pressure.

Annuloplasty: Surgical reduction in the size of the annulus to reduce or eliminate valvular regurgitation. Generally performed on mitral and tricuspid valves.

Annulus: A fibrous structure to which the valve leaflets are attached; it serves as a hinge.

Anticoagulant: Agent used to thin the blood.

Anticoagulation: Process of thinning the blood using medication such as heparin or warfarin.

Aorta: The artery transporting blood from the left ventricle to the rest of the body through its various branches.

Aortic dissection: A tear in the wall of the aorta, which may be life threatening, due to aortic rupture. Common causes are hypertension, Marfan syndrome, and conditions causing weakening of arterial wall.

Aortic regurgitation: A leaky aortic valve such that blood leaks back from the aorta to the left ventricle.

Aortic root: Part of the ascending aorta immediately above the aortic valve.

Aortic stenosis: Narrowing of the aortic valve such that the left ventricle has to generate a higher pressure to pump blood.

Aortic valve: A trileaflet valve between the left ventricle and aorta. This prevents blood from leaking back into the left ventricle from the aorta.

Arrhythmia: Abnormal rhythm that may be too slow or too fast. Examples include heart block and atrial fibrillation.

Atrial fibrillation: A rhythm disorder in which the atria quiver instead of contracting. This can predispose to blood clots inside the atria and increase stroke risk and erratic heart rate response. It generally occurs because of enlarged atria, which can occur with valvular problems.

Atrium: One of two upper chambers that receives blood; the right atrium receives blood from the body and the left atrium receives it from the lungs.

Autograft: A valve from one's own body. For example, in a Ross procedure, a patient's own pulmonary valve (autograft) is used to replace a diseased aortic valve. The excised pulmonary valve is replaced by a homograft.

Bacteria: Microorganisms with a cell wall. The body has many bacteria on the skin, oral cavity, and intestines that do not cause any harm. Sometimes they cause harm, such as infection, on the heart valves. Examples include streptococci and staphylococci.

Beta-blocker: A medication that blocks the beta receptor, which is a receptor for adrenaline and noradrena-

line. The beta-blockers slow the heart rate and lower the blood pressure. They are also protective in patients with heart attacks and heart failure.

Bicuspid: A valve made of two valve leaflets.

Bioprosthesis: An artificial valve made of animal or human tissue. It could be a porcine or bovine valve, a valve made of pericardium or a valve harvested from another human being postmortem. A human cadaveric derived valve is called a homograft.

Bleeding: Blood getting outside the blood vessels, generally because of damage to vessels or heart chambers.

Carcinoid syndrome: A hormone-secreting tumor manifesting with flushing, diarrhea, and valvular problems mostly affecting the right side of the heart.

Cardiac: Related to the heart.

Cardiac catheterization: Inserting a catheter into the heart through a peripheral artery or a vein to record the pressures or obtain an angiogram or intervene to fix a lesion.

Cardiomyopathy: Heart muscle disease. Broadly, there are four types: dilated, hypertrophic, restrictive, and obliterative.

Chordae tendinae: Stringlike structures that support mitral and tricuspid valves.

Congenital: Something one is born with.

Congestive heart failure: *See* heart failure.

Coumadin: *See* warfarin.

Degenerative: Change produced by wear and tear.

Deoxygenated: Blood from which oxygen is removed and used up by tissues.

Diastole: Phase of the cardiac cycle during which the ventricles are not contracting. The ventricles fill with blood during this period.

Dilated cardiomyopathy: Heart muscle disease that causes dilation and weakening of the heart muscle leading to heart failure. Outcome is improved by beta-blockers and angiotensin converting enzyme inhibitors.

Doppler: An ultrasound examination of the heart based on Doppler principle. This allows visualization of flow and measurement of blood flow velocities.

Dyspnea: Shortness of breath. *See* paroxysmal nocturnal dyspnea.

Ebstein's anomaly: A congenital malformation of the tricuspid valve with apical displacement of one of its leaflets causing tricuspid regurgitation. This can be associated with arrhythmias as well.

Echocardiography: Examination of the heart using ultrasound. One can obtain images of the heart and examine blood flows.

Embolus: A solid particle that gets dislodged from one part of the circulation to another. Commonly, it is a thrombus (thromboembolism), less frequently an atheroma, piece of a tumor, vegetation, or air bubble.

Endocarditis: Inflammation of the valve or inner lining of the heart generally due to infection such as streptococcus or staphylococcus.

Endocardium: Inner lining of the heart.

Eustachian valve: A vestigial valve between the inferior vena cava and the right atrium with no known functions in adult life. In the intrauterine life, this directs umbilical vein flow into the left atrium through the patent foramen ovale.

Fen-Phen: A combination of weight-loss drugs used in the 1990s that caused valvular problems. This drug was taken off the market with a large class-action lawsuit.

Flail valve: Loss of support to the valve, generally due to torn chordae tendinae, causing valvular regurgitation. It can affect the mitral or tricuspid valve.

Functional regurgitation: Valve regurgitation with intrinsically normal leaflets. Causes may be dilated annulus or tethered leaflets.

Fungus (*plural:* fungi): A microorganism that can cause endocarditis.

Heart failure: A situation where demand on the heart exceeds its capacity. It generally occurs due to weakening of the heart muscle or a severe valve problem. Manifestations include shortness of breath, swelling in the legs, fatigue, and swollen neck veins.

Holter monitor: A device for continuous monitoring of the heartbeat to detect arrhythmia. Generally this is worn for 24-48 hrs and when symptoms occur, the patient can store the recording by pressing a button.

Homograft: Valve from a human cadaver used to replace a diseased valve in a patient.

Hypertrophy: Thickening of the wall of the heart due to more muscle mass.

Infarction: Death of heart muscle due to lack of blood supply

Inferior vena cava: A large vein that drains impure blood from the lower part of the body into the right atrium.

Inflammation: Literally means setting fire. Medically, it is a body's response to any invasion. It is protective, but it can cause damage as well. Cardinal features of inflammation are pain, redness, swelling, heat, and loss of function. Endocarditis and rheumatic fever are examples of inflammation.

International normalized ratio (INR): Method used to measure how thin the blood is and to adjust a dose of warfarin.

Ischemia: Reduced blood supply causing lack of oxygen to the tissues.

Ischemic mitral regurgitation: Mitral regurgitation that is caused by a heart attack or ischemic weakening and dilatation of the heart muscle.

Marfan syndrome: A genetic disorder causing weakening of connective tissue. Features include tall stature, dislocation of ocular lens, valve prolapse, and aortic aneurysm.

Mechanical valve: An artificial valve with metallic components. These need to be anticoagulated.

Median sternotomy: A type of surgical procedure in which a vertical inline incision is made along the sternum, after which the sternum itself is divided, or "cracked."

Migraine: A throbbing headache thought to be related to excessive dilation of the blood vessels in the brain due to some circulating substance. There is an association with patent foramen ovale and mitral valve prolapse.

Minimally invasive: A surgery performed without a large scar; it could be robotically assisted.

Mitral regurgitation: Leaky mitral valve such that blood leaks back from the left ventricle into the left atrium.

Mitral stenosis: Narrowed mitral valve such that the left atrial pressure rises in order to push blood forward, from the left atrium to the left ventricle.

Mitral valve: A bileaflet valve separating the left atrium and left ventricle.

Murmur: A noise produced by flowing blood that can be heard with a stethoscope. Some noises could be normal, but louder ones and diastolic ones are generally abnormal.

Myxomatous: Thickened, fluffy, weaker tissue as may occur in mitral valve prolapse.

Orthopnea: Shortness of breath relieved by sitting up; this is a feature of heart failure.

Oxygenated: Replenished with oxygen, e.g., blood that is replenished with oxygen by the lungs.

Pallor: Pale skin color. This can occur because of anemia or low blood count.

Palpitations: Feeling one's own heartbeat. This could be either benign or abnormal.

Papillary muscle: A muscle bundle inside the heart that anchors chordae tendinae into the ventricular wall. The left ventricle has two and the right ventricle has three.

Paroxysmal nocturnal dyspnea: Intermittent shortness of breath that typically wakes the patient up from sleep at night. Is a sign of left-side heart failure.

Prolapse: Excessive systolic motion of a cardiac valve due to loss of support.

Prophylaxis: A measure used to prevent disease.

Prosthetic valve: Artificial valve made of tissue or metal.

Pulmonary artery: The artery that transports blood from the right ventricle to the lungs.

Pulmonary regurgitation: Leaky pulmonary valve such that blood leaks back from the pulmonary artery into the right ventricle.

Pulmonary stenosis: Narrowing of the pulmonary valve such that the right ventricle has to generate a higher pressure to pump blood into the lungs.

Pulmonary valve: The trileaflet valve between the right ventricle and the pulmonary artery.

Pulmonary vein: A thin walled blood vessel that brings oxygenated blood from the lungs into the left atrium. There are four pulmonary veins, two from each lung.

Regurgitation: Leaky valve.

Reverse remodeling: A favorable change in which the heart size gets smaller.

Rheumatic fever: Fever that may occur after streptococcal infections, resulting in joint pains, skin lesions, and inflammation of the heart. Inflammation of the heart results in valvular problems.

Ross procedure: A surgical procedure in which a patient's own pulmonary valve is used to replace the aortic valve and a homograft is used to replace the explanted pulmonary valve.

Stenosis: Narrowing of a valve or a blood vessel.

Stroke: Damage to part of the brain due a blockage in the artery or bleeding.

Superior vena cava: Vena cava or large vein that drains blood from the upper part of the body into the right atrium.

Systole: Phase of the cardiac cycle during which the ventricles contract and pump blood.

Tethering: Restricted systolic mobility of valve leaflets because of being pulled down by chordae tendinae.

Tetralogy of Fallot: A congenital cyanotic (blue skin color because of low oxygen content) heart disease consisting of pulmonary stenosis, large ventricular septal defect, right ventricular hypertrophy, and aorta overriding the ventricular septal defect.

Transthoracic echocardiogram: A standard, noninvasive echocardiogram where a transducer records the sound wave echoes of the heart as they reflect off internal structures.

Tricuspid regurgitation: Leaky tricuspid valve such that blood leaks back from the right ventricle into the right atrium.

Tricuspid stenosis: Narrowing of the tricuspid valve such that the right atrial pressure rises to push blood across the stenosed valve.

Tricuspid valve: The trileaflet valve between the right atrium and the right ventricle.

Ultrasound: Sound wave above the hearing range (> 20,000 Hz) used to perform echocardiography.

Valve: A structure made of two or three leaflets designed to allow blood to flow in one direction only. There are four valves inside the heart—mitral, aortic, tricuspid, and pulmonary.

Valvuloplasty: Opening up a stenosed valve with a balloon, a device, or surgically.

Vegetation: An inflammatory mass attached to a valve, endocardium, or endothelium. This is most commonly due to an infection and most commonly occurs on a heart valve.

Vena cava: One of the two large veins that drain impure blood from the body into the right atrium.

Ventricle: Lower chamber of the heart that pumps blood into an artery. The left ventricle pumps into the aorta. The right ventricle pumps into the pulmonary artery, which takes blood into the lungs to be oxygenated.

Warfarin: Blood thinner taken orally. It blocks the effect of vitamin K and works on the liver. This prevents blood clots on the mechanical valves and those in atrial fibrillation.

Xenograft: An artificial or prosthetic valve made of animal tissue.

Index